DEFENDING THE AGING BRAIN

FIGHT COGNITIVE DECLINE, AGE GRACEFULLY USING THESE 5 SIMPLE STEPS, AND ACQUIRE A HEALTHY, POWERFUL MIND

WALTER BISHOP

CONTENTS

INTRODUCTION

The brain is the most complex, challenging scientific puzzle we have ever tried to decode.

— PAUL ALLEN, CO-FOUNDER OF
MICROSOFT

People like Jennifer Lopez, the American singer, actress, and dancer age in reverse as evidenced through their photos, among other things. When Lopez was 50 years old, she hosted Saturday Night Live (SNL) and emphasized that she was growing backward (Eight Saints, n.d.). Although her age in number is increasing, Lopez's skin, outlook, and business acumen do not seem to follow suit. It's never too late for you to reverse or pause the aging process. More importantly, we will share some tips in this book about how you can slow down the rate at which your brain ages.

Do you often feel like you need to quickly do something to delay your brain from aging so that your children will not see you as a burden? Could it be that you sometimes think about how your aging brain might affect your functionality as years go by? You might be anxious that cognitive decline will see you being displaced from your position at work by younger employees. If you have ever tried to get information about cognitive decline from the internet, you might have realized how difficult gathering the relevant details might be. This is because the information on internet sources is usually so scattered therefore, picking the right pieces is quite tedious. If you can relate to any of these questions and statements, please know that you are not alone. Moreover, this book is a specific compilation of everything that you need to know with regard to taking good care of your brain and staying away from triggers that quicken its deterioration as you age.

PILLARS OF GOOD BRAIN HEALTH

There are many things you can do to ensure that your brain ages gracefully. Here is an overview of some pillars for good brain health as we will discuss in various chapters of this book:

- **Physical exercise:** Physical exercise has undisputable benefits for your brain. Your ability to learn, think, control emotions, and logically solve problems improves when you exercise.
- **Food and nutrition:** Lopez and other celebrities who are admired for their ever-young brains, are selective when it comes to what they eat. They prefer food that builds up their mental resilience while staying away from those that can harm them.
- **Sleep and relaxation:** Your body and brain also need to rest sometimes. Overworking your brain and depriving it of periods of relaxation will exhaust its energy and make it susceptible to cognitive decline. Sleep rejuvenates your brain.
- **Mental fitness:** Your brain needs to work out, in the same way your physical body does.

Learning and engaging in genuine relationships contribute to better mental fitness.

- **Social interaction:** A wide and healthy social network contributes to your physical, emotional, and psychological well-being. The people around you can provide you with support, thereby, reducing your risk of stress, anxiety, and depression, all of which trigger faster cognitive decline. Aim to create positive interactions at work, home, in your community, and beyond.

BENEFITS OF MAINTAINING YOUR BRAIN

You could be asking, "Suppose I take good care of my brain, what's in it for me?" We will answer this question for you here. A few of the benefits that come with maintaining your brain health the proper way are:

- **Improved brain functions:** Your brain can be divided into two sections, the right and left brain hemispheres. The left side of the brain is the one that is responsible for calculations, reading, and writing abilities. The right side is highly visual so it mainly deals with images and creativity. Ensuring that your brain is healthy will improve all the brain functions that are related to each hemisphere. Learning numbers and language becomes easier.

- **Quicker reaction time:** A healthier brain correlates with quicker reaction time. Your brain is receiving the information and processing it more efficiently. As a result, you complete tasks at a faster rate. Your confidence in completing tasks also improves.
- **Increases audio and visual abilities:** The brain also controls your sight, hearing, and other senses. If you want your senses to be more acute and effective, take proper care of your brain.
- **Gives you more confidence:** People who are emotionally stable, accompanied by healthier bodily functions tend to exhibit better self-esteem. The same happens when the reaction time and rate of successful task completion are higher. In essence, good brain health elevates your overall self-confidence.
- **Improve bodily functions:** Your brain is responsible for regulating some functions in your body, including blood circulation, breathing, and processing information. When your brain is healthier, these bodily functions are more efficient.

- **Delay cognitive decline:** Thinking and recalling abilities are enhanced when your brain is healthier. The healthier your brain, the longer you will retain your critical thinking processes.

SUPER-AGERS

Have you ever heard of super-agers? These are individuals who do not seem to exhibit the usual effects of an aging brain. They just can't forget facts they saw before, unlike their agemates who may forget within moments. They still successfully complete puzzles, even at 85 years of age. The memory of super-agers is laser-sharp. One study that investigated the super-agers found that they have lower numbers of *fiber-like tangles* in their brains, compared to their counterparts who age normally (Paul, 2008). Tangles are made up of a protein called "tau" and it progressively accumulates in the brain, eventually destroying the cells. Therefore, the fewer the tangles, the higher the chances that your brain cells can remain healthy. The researchers also brought forward the notion that some people are immune to the formation of tangles, which makes them super-agers.

In another study, two mechanisms for protection from age-related mental illnesses were reported (Singer,

2021). These are resilience and resistance. Those who are resistant completely do not go through the typical pathology that is associated with cognitive decline. On the other hand, resilient individuals experience the pathology that is linked to aging, but they do not exhibit signs of dementia. This means that there is hope for better cognitive health, even when pathological signs of aging catch up with you. In this book, we will share with you some of the tips on how to become resilient against age-related brain issues.

GET READY TO START!

Apart from Lopez, other Hollywood stars who seem to defy the power of aging are Kim Kardashian, Jennifer Aniston, Halle Berry, and Gwen Stefani. You can enjoy the benefits of maintaining your brain, like these celebrities, if you follow the information that will be revealed in this book. Fasten your belt and start your journey toward long-term, if not life-long cognitive health!

1

THE BRAIN

This chapter talks about the brain as one of the body's main organs and memory as the most commonly recognized cognitive function. Let's kick it off by talking about Peter Green's story. Green was a white male who was in his late '80s and was a participant in longitudinal studies that focused on the elderly at the University of California San Francisco (UCSF) Memory and Aging Center. Joel Kramer, a neuropsychologist who assessed Green's brain reported that they were no different from those of the other senior citizens who were involved in this study. After scanning Green's brain, Kramer described them as "not pretty" (UCSF, n.d.). The researcher even observed patches of dead matter throughout Green's white matter. This showed that the participant had experienced some ministrokes that usually come with cognitive decline.

Normally, the observations that were made on Green's brain would correlate with notable cognitive decline as is often the case in many people of his age. Surprisingly for Green, the opposite was true, his functioning ability remained very high and his cognitive test results were excellent. An even more interesting investigation, according to Kramer, was that Green's high cognition and impeccable functioning level remained constant over a period of years. After a one-on-one encounter with Green, Kramer realized that Green had a very open, grateful, and joyous approach to life. He remained connected to the community and his family as much as he could. Green embraced building and maintaining good relationships while making sure that he doesn't allow minor issues to stress him. Green is a great example of a super-ager. You could be the next super-ager of your time!

BRAIN ANATOMY

The brain is among the most complex organs that you have as a human being. This organ regulates various functionalities in your body, including breathing, emotions, hunger, vision, memory, thought, and touch. The brain is a major component of the central nervous system (CNS), together with the spinal cord. You might be wondering what makes up this organ that weighs approximately three pounds in adults. Surprisingly, 60% of the brain is made up of fat. Carbohydrates, water, salts, and proteins make up the remaining 40% of this vital organ You will also find glial cells, neurons, and blood vessels in the brain. Please note that the brain on its own can't be referred to as a "muscle."

The White and Gray Matter

The white and gray matter describes two regions that are found in the CNS. Remember, we mentioned that the CNS is made up of the brain and the spinal cord earlier on. In the brain, the gray matter is the darker region that occupies an area of the organ. The inner section of the brain is lighter and this is what is referred to as the "white" matter. When it comes to the spinal cord, the white matter is the one that occupies the outer surface while the gray matter is the inner space.

For you to understand the gray and white matter more, we will talk about the anatomy of neurons in brief. Neurons consist of three parts: which are the round central cell bodies, axons, and dendrites. You could visualize these components in the form of a tree with branches (dendrites), trunk (cell bodies), and roots (axon) (Woodruff, 2016).

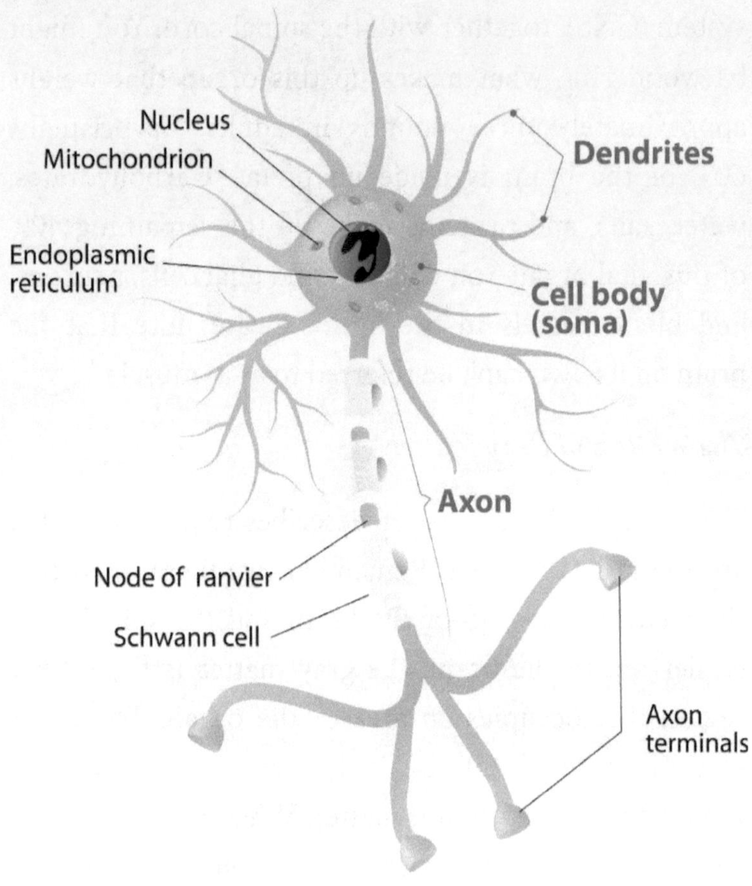

The cell body is also known as the "soma" and this is where the nucleus (center) of the neuron is located. This means that the soma contains the DNA and that's where proteins are translated. The dendrites are the point of contact between the neuron and other cells. In other words, communication with other cells takes place through the dendrites. The axon is a long stem that connects neurons to each other and it is covered with a myelin sheath, which is a protective coating.

The gray matter is mainly made up of the neuron somas while axons are the major nerve component in the white matter. This neuronal composition explains why the white and gray matter appears in different shades under a scan. The gray and white matter also have different functions. Information is processed and interpreted in gray matter. The white matter is responsible for transmitting the processed information to the rest of the nervous system. This also explains why the axons abundantly exist in the white matter.

OTHER MAIN PARTS OF THE BRAIN

The brain works by sending and receiving electrical and chemical signals to and from different parts of the brain. These signals work with the brain to regulate various functions and processes in your body. For instance, when you feel a pain sensation, these brain signals are sending and receiving information such as the location and severity of the injury. Please note that not all signals are transmitted to various parts of your body. Some information is retained within the brain. All these functions of the brain are made possible by the neurons. The brain is also divided into different parts that have separate responsibilities that together aid the overall function of the brain. We will discuss these brain components, including the brain stem, cerebrum, and cerebellum in this section.

Cerebrum

The cerebrum is the largest part of the brain and is known as the "front of the brain." It has both white and gray matter. Judgment, problem-solving, speech, learning, thinking, and emotions are some of the functions that are regulated by the cerebrum. This region of the brain also controls important senses such as hearing, vision, and touch. Apart from regulating temperature, the cerebrum is also responsible for initiating and coordinating your movements.

The cerebral cortex is the gray matter covering of the cerebrum. The cerebral cortex is folded in layers so it covers a huge surface area. This also explains why this part makes up approximately half of the overall weight of the brain. The cortex is made up of two hemispheres, with the one on the right side controlling the left side of the body and vice versa. The two halves of the cerebral cortex do not work independently. They communicate with each other through the corpus callosum, which is a structure that is made up of white matter and nerve pathways. The two hemispheres of the cerebral cortex join at the point known as the "sulcus" that stretches from the front of your head to the back.

Brain Stem

This is the middle of the brain, being the link between the cerebrum and spinal cord. There are three components that make up the brain stem and these are the midbrain, medulla, and pons. Please note that the midbrain is also called the mesencephalon. It is complex and is made up of neural pathways, and neuron clusters, among other structures. When you calculate responses and environmental changes, it's your midbrain at work. This part of the brain is also involved in other functions such as hearing and movement. The substantia nigra and basal ganglia make it possible for the midbrain to deal with movement and coordination.

The pons mark the point where four of the twelve cranial nerves originate. Cranial nerves play an important role in focusing your vision, producing tears, blinking, chewing, facial expressions, and balance. The *pons*—which is the Latin term for "bridge"—connect the midbrain to the medulla. The brain meets the spinal cord at a point that is known as the medulla. This part of the brain is responsible for functions that aid your everyday survival. The major roles carried out by the medulla include controlling breathing, heart rate, blood flow, as well as carbon dioxide and oxygen levels in your body. In order to control such bodily functions, the medulla aids reflexive functions that include, but are not limited to, coughing, sneezing, and vomiting.

Cerebellum

The term "little brain" is sometimes used to refer to the cerebellum. This component is located at the back of the brain, slightly above the brain stem, and its size compares to that of a fist. The cerebellum also consists of two hemispheres. The outer region of the cerebellum contains neurons. Communication with the cerebral cortex takes place in the inner region. Coordination of voluntary muscle movements, as well as balance, posture, and equilibrium maintenance, are all functions of the cerebellum. It is thought that the cerebellum might be involved in regulating thoughts, emotions, and social behaviors. These notions are being investigated through scientific experiments by scientists (John Hopkins Medicine, 2019).

Brain Coverings

Being a delicate organ, the brain is protected by three layers of covering, called the meninges. These meninges also surround the spinal cord. Simply put, the meninges describe a set of three membranes that line the skull with the main responsibility of protecting the brain. These three membranes are the pia mater, arachnoid, and dura mater.

- **Pia mater:** The pia mater is the one that directly covers the surface of the brain. It is a very thin membrane allowing it to smoothly follow over the contours of the brain as it protects the organ. Veins and arteries are contained in the pia mater.
- **Arachnoid membrane:** The arachnoid membrane is thin, and resembles a web in appearance. Blood vessels and nerves are not found in this layer. Immediately below the arachnoid membrane, you will find the cerebrospinal fluid (CSF), which apart from cushioning the brain and spinal cord, also continuously removes impurities from these organs.
- **Dura mater:** The dura mater is the outermost layer of the meninges. Unlike the other two innermost membranes, the dura mater is thicker and stronger. There are two layers that make up the dura mater and these are the periosteal and meningeal layers. The periosteal layer is the one that is in direct contact with the inner side of the skull while the meningeal layer is located right below it. Please note that there are also spaces between these two layers of the dura mater. The purpose of these spaces is to

allow blood vessels to pass through as they control blood flow to and from the brain.

Lobes of the Brain

To enhance effective function, the brain is divided into sections that have specific responsibilities. These sections are found in each hemisphere of the brain and they are called lobes. The brain has four lobes in total, namely temporal, frontal, occipital, and parietal. Let's explore more about these lobes in this section.

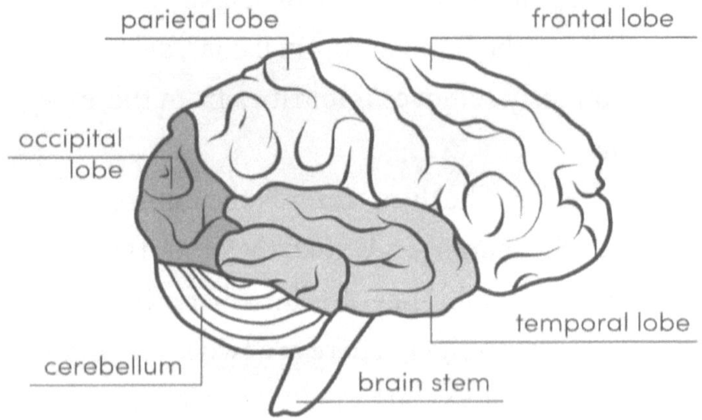

- **Frontal lobe:** This is the largest lobe and as its name suggests, it is found at the front of the head. Functions that are associated with movement, personality traits, and decision-making are controlled by the frontal lobe. The Broca's area, which is involved in enhancing speech ability, is located within the frontal lobe. Parts of the frontal lobe also contribute to smell recognition.

- **Occipital lobe:** This lobe is located at the back of your brain. It is involved in vision functionalities.
- **Temporal lobe:** The temporal lobe makes up the sides of the brain. This lobe enhances musical rhythm, short-term memory, and speech. It also, to some extent, contributes to smell recognition.
- **Parietal lobe:** This marks the middle region of your brain. Your ability to identify objects is enhanced by this part of the brain. Spatial relationships, which involve comparison between your body and objects that surround it, are also controlled by the parietal lobe of the brain. Detecting and interpreting touch and pain is made possible by this lobe. Your ability to understand spoken language is enhanced by the Wernicke's area, which is located in the parietal lobe.

Deeper Brain Structures

The brain also has other structures that enhance its overall functions. These include the hypothalamus, hippocampus, amygdala, as well as pituitary, and pineal glands. In this section, we will discuss more of these crucial brain structures.

▷ Hippocampus

This organ assumes a sea-horse shape. It is located under the temporal lobes. For it to perform its functions, the hippocampus gets information from the cerebral cortex. It is reported that this organ plays a vital role in Alzheimer's disease. The hippocampus supports your learning, memory, and navigation abilities.

▷ Pineal Gland

Located deep within the brain is the pineal gland. This gland is highly responsive to light changes and darkness. The pineal gland is the one that produces melatonin, the hormone that regulates the sleep-wake cycle and the Circadian rhythms.

▷ Hypothalamus

The hypothalamus works hand-in-hand with the pituitary gland, which probably explains why the two are located close to each other. The hypothalamus sends chemical messages to the pituitary gland, thereby controlling the latter's functions. The hypothalamus is involved in controlling hunger, thirst, and temperatures. It also plays a crucial role in synchronizing sleep patterns, in addition to regulating emotion and memory functions.

▷ Pituitary Gland

The pituitary gland is the size of a pea and it is located behind the bridge of the nose. This gland controls the functions of other glands in your body, which explain why it is also referred to as the "master gland." Simply put, the flow of hormones from the ovaries, thyroid, testicles, and adrenals is controlled by the pituitary gland. For this gland to carry out its functions, it receives messages from the hypothalamus via the blood supply or its stalk.

▷ Amygdala

The amygdala is located below both hemispheres of the brain. It is a small structure that has the shape of an almond. It takes part in regulating your memory and emotions. The "fight or flight" response that happens when you perceive a threat, is also controlled by the amygdala. This structure also controls the reward system for your brain.

▷ Ventricles and Cerebrospinal Fluids

The brain also contains four open spaces that have passages. These open areas connect to the central spinal canal. The CSF is made in the ventricles. The main role of the CSF is to serve as a cushion that protects the spinal cord and brain. It is also the medium through which nutrients are transported to these organs. The CSF also removes impurities and waste that is made through the various processes that take place in the brain.

THE BRAIN AND BLOOD SUPPLY

For the brain to survive, there has to be a way for it to receive blood from the heart. Apparently, there are two sets of blood vessels whose responsibility is to ensure blood and oxygen supply to the brain. These are the carotid arteries and vertebral arteries. If you have ever tried to feel your pulse through the side of your neck, then you were dealing with the external carotid arteries. The internal carotid arteries supply blood to the front part of the brain.

The vertebral arteries stretch along the spinal column and enter the skull. When they reach the brain stem, the arteries form what is called the basilar artery. This is the one that supplies blood to the back of the brain. Close to the bottom of the brain, there is a loop of blood vessels that is known as the circle of Willis. This is the point where major blood vessels connect. The circle of Willis ensures efficient supply and circulation of blood from the front to the back region of the brain.

It makes it possible for various arteries to interact with each other.

THE CRANIAL NERVES

The cranium is the dome of the skull and it harbors 12 different nerves, which are referred to as the cranial nerves. These nerves are the focus in this section. Please note that two of the cranial nerves that we will discuss, which are the olfactory and optic nerves, emerge from the cerebrum. The rest of the nerves have their origins in the brain stem. Going through this section will assist you to see the extent to which the brain is vastly involved with other parts of your body.

- **The olfactory nerve:** This nerve enhances your sense of smell.
- **The optic nerve:** This is responsible for eyesight.
- **The oculomotor nerve:** This nerve deals with various movements by the eye, including those of the pupil.
- **The trochlear nerve:** Various muscles in the eyes are controlled by this nerve.
- **The trigeminal nerve:** This nerve takes part in sensory and motor functions. Chewing muscles are also controlled by the trigeminal nerve. This

nerve is not only the largest among the cranial nerves, but it is also the most complex.

- **The abducens nerve:** This is the source of nerves for some muscles in your eyes.
- **The facial nerve:** The functions of the facial nerve include taste, face movement, and glandular functions.
- **The vestibulocochlear nerve:** This nerve is involved in balance and hearing.
- **The glossopharyngeal nerve:** Some of the functions of the nerve are enabling throat and ear movement, as well as enhancing the sense of taste.
- **The vagus nerve:** The motor activity in the digestive system, heart, and throat is controlled by this nerve. The vagus nerve is also responsible for all sensations that involve your ears.
- **The accessory nerve:** This nerve deals with specific muscles that are found in the shoulder, neck, and head.
- **The hypoglossal nerve:** This is the nerve that is responsible for supplying the tongue with motor activity.

MEMORY, THE MOTHER OF ALL WISDOM

Memory describes all psychological processes that involve gathering, storing, preserving, and redeeming information. In scientific terms, creating memories involves strengthening already-existing connections between neurons or forming completely new connections that weren't there before (NIH, n.d.). This probably explains why going through information many times makes it easier for you to remember it.

Memories can be classified according to how long they last. Memories that are associated with sensory signals about the world are usually very brief. They last for a few seconds. Some memories last for about 30 seconds and these are described as short-term. Short-term memories apply when you are focusing on something, even a task. They could refer to thoughts that might just be passing through your mind. In some cases, memories can stretch up to days, months, years, decades, or even a lifetime. Such memories are termed "long-term memories" because they stick around for longer.

Stages of Memory Creation

The concept of memory is well explained using three processes, which are encoding, storage, and retrieval (Cherry, 2020). The formation of new memories begins with the process of encoding. This is when the gathered information is converted into a form that is usable, prior to storing it to later use. We will further explore the three stages of memory in this section.

▷ Encoding

Encoding describes the first encounter of gathering, perceiving, and learning information. Simply put, encoding involves making sense of available or provided information. Suppose you just see people running out of a building while some are screaming. If you then see some smoke coming out through the building's opening, what deductions are you going to make? Whether you assume that there has been a fire outbreak or what, the fact is that you would have used the information that you would have gathered to make sense of the situation. That is encoding.

▷ Storage

Each encounter you have in your life will impact some changes. Upon each experience, you gather some information which is then stored in your mind. Explaining this deeper, the information that you encode causes changes in the nervous system and this creates new impressions. Every new impression comes with changes in your brain. It is these changes that enhance the storage of memories.

▷ **Retrieval**

Some experts argue that the main stage as far as memory is concerned is retrieval (McDermott, 2013). The reason for this is relatively straightforward. What is the use of information that is encoded and stored, if it cannot be retrieved? Interestingly, most of the information that you encode will never be consciously retrieved. However, the ability to access the stored information when necessary is very important.

Memory Creation and Time

Creating memories can be described in terms of time progression. As time elapses, memories transform from sensory register, to short-term memory, and then to long-term memory. Let's delve deeper into these concepts.

▷ **Sensory Register**

During sensory registering, your brain gathers information from the world around you. The sensory register is a process that does not take more than a few seconds. This stage of memory creation is usually passive, which is why it is also called 'echoic' memory. Think of what happens when you ask a presenter to repeat a statement that they would have said before. You would have heard what they said the first time but in an 'echoic' manner. The moment you pay more attention to information during the sensory register, then you begin to transition to short-term memory. Therefore, attention is regarded as the stage that separates the sensory register and short-term memory.

▷ Short-Term Memory

Short-term memory can be explained in two ways. First, there is what has always been known as "short-term" memory. This form is when the information is temporarily stored for the purposes of repeating it. If someone gives you their address, you are more likely to use short-term memory for you to remember it. Second, there is working memory. In this case, the information is stored so that you can manipulate it. Solving a math problem will require working memory.

▷ Long-Term Memory

With long-term memory, information can be stored in your brain for an indefinite period of time. For long-term memories to be formed, the information from the working memory is retrieved by the hippocampus. This information is then used to physically transform the neural wiring in your brain. The new connections that would have been developed remained for as long as possible.

Long-term memory can be classified according to the nature of the memories involved. This form of classification will divide long-term memory into explicit or implicit memory.

- **Implicit memories** are the ones that you remember automatically.
- **Explicit memories** are the ones that involve conscious effort on your part for you to remember them. Explicit mores are further divided into episodic and semantic memories. Episodic ones are those that happen to you as an individual. They are so specific and direct, unlike the semantic memories that involve general knowledge.

Memory and Brain Parts

You could be wondering if creating and storing memories involves just one part of the brain or not. The purpose of this section is to respond to your thoughts and provide you with relevant information. Basically, different parts of the brain are involved when it comes to memory.

▷ The Amygdala

The amygdala is responsible for controlling emotions such as fear. Emotions like aggression and fear promote the secretion of stress hormones. These hormones are largely involved in the storage of memories. The amygdala's involvement in processing emotional information enhances the consolidation of memory. In other words, the amygdala enhances your ability to transform newly learned information into long-term memory. It makes it easy for you to remember things that involve some emotional connection.

▷ The Hippocampus

According to research the hippocampus plays a vital role in memory (Spielman et al., 2014). The results showed that this organ is mainly involved in spatial memory and normal recognition memory. Additionally, the hippocampus also provides information to cortical regions of the brain. This process is important for attaching meaning to memories as they get connected to other established ones. Like the amygdala, the hippocampus is also involved in memory consolidation. If your hippocampus gets injured, you lose the ability to create new memories.

▷ The Prefrontal Cortex and Cerebellum

From what you have learned so far, it is clear that the hippocampus is involved in creating explicit memories. The cerebellum, on the other hand, helps you to create implicit ones. Often known as non-declarative memory, implicit memory is the one that does not need you to consciously recollect information from past events. You can think of implicit memory as procedural. Results from positron emission tomography (PET) revealed that the prefrontal cortex plays a role in processing and preserving information (Spielman et al., 2014).

▷ Neurotransmitters

Neurons secrete chemical substances used to affect other cells across a gap that is known as the synapse. These chemical substances are called neurotransmitters and their roles in memory are of paramount importance. Some of the neurotransmitters that are worth mentioning are serotonin, epinephrine, acetylcholine, and dopamine. The communication between neurons, as enhanced by neurotransmitters, is crucial in memory creation and retention. As neurons continue to act, more neurotransmitters are released into the synapses. Memory consolidation happens as the synapses are triggered.

The secretion of neurotransmitters is also associated with the emotional characteristics of the information involved. When an event is associated with stronger emotional feelings, memories are more likely to be retained for longer. The opposite is also true. When you get stressed, you will release more of the neurotransmitter called glutamate. This is why you rarely forget stressful situations in life.

THE CONCEPT OF FORGETTING

Even when our brains are designed to maintain memory, there are times when we forget things. The tendency of forgetting seems to worsen with age. However, forgetting can take place simply because of the inability to pay enough attention to information. In some cases, it may be due to the failure of the brain to consolidate information. Two concepts, the decaying and interference theories are often used to explain forgetting.

The Decaying Theory

The decay theory is based on the fact that memory can just disappear as time progresses. In other words, memory is more available for retrieval soon after it has been stored than later. Another explanation to decay theory is that memory strength reduces with time. This is why it is recommended that you constantly rehearse information for it to remain available for retrieval. Another important point to note is that the decay theory mainly targets short-term memory, rather than long-term.

The Interference Theory

The interference theory suggests that long-term and short-term memory hamper each other. Therefore, it is impossible for information that is stored in long-term memory to be retrieved into short-term memory. Remember, short-term memory involves a temporal workspace so retrieving specific memories that had been previously stored as long-term memory can be difficult. Think of how difficult it can be for you to remember an old password after you have created a new one. That is the interference theory at play.

THE FAILURES OF MEMORY

You have at some point in life experienced the failures that are associated with memory. Let's discuss some of the common memory failures that you might relate to within this section.

- **Bias:** This describes a situation where your current or previous beliefs, thoughts, and knowledge interfere with your memory system.
- **Transience:** This is a time-related scenario where memories just become less accessible as time elapses. Transience is usually due to aging processes, as well as injury or damage to parts of the brain, especially the hippocampus.
- **Suggestibility:** When misinformation becomes incorporated into your memory, you have a scenario of failure due to suggestibility. A good

example is when you are asked a leading question.

- **Persistence:** Some memories are simply difficult to get past, no matter how much you try. Persistence describes this phenomenon where some memories continue to stick around your mind.
- **Blocking:** Blocking is also referred to as the "tip of the tongue" syndrome. It is when memories become temporarily inaccessible. An example of this frustrating memory failure is trying to recall the name of an acquaintance.
- **Misattribution:** This happens when memories cannot be confirmed for some reason. For instance, if you cannot trust the source of the information that you got, misattribution takes place.
- **Absent-mindedness:** This is when you simply lose focus and attention on what you are doing. You might even forget tasks in the process, like walking into a room and forgetting why you were going there..

THE STORY OF PHINEAS GAGE

Have you ever heard of the man who founded neuroscience, Phineas Gage? This man survived an accident during which an iron rod went through his skull. Much of the frontal lobe of his brain was damaged in the process. Soon after the accident, Gage's personality changed completely such that even his close friends noticed. Gage's behavior change helped neuroscientists to have an idea of the important responsibilities of the brain's frontal lobe, especially in association with personalities. Before the accident, Gage was known to be hardworking and focused on his work. After the unfortunate incident, he became an alcoholic who could not keep his job.

After studying Gage's brain, researchers found out that the prefrontal cortices of the brain were severely affected. This had the effect of altering Gage's emotional command and ability to make decisions.

FUN FACTS ABOUT YOUR BRAIN

There are many things that you might find interesting as far as your brain is concerned. Here are some facts that are with noting:

- **Information in the brain travels at a speed of 268 miles per hour:** The information travels in the form of electrical impulses from one cell to another.

- **The total weight of the human brain is three pounds:** This weight can be equated to half a gallon of milk. Generally, men have bigger brains than women. Please note that the size of the brain does not correlate to intelligence.
- **A brain tissue piece whose size is equal to that of a grain of sand has 100,000 neurons and a billion synapses:** This explains why seemingly small damage to the brain may have a negative impact on its health. Many neurons and synapses are disturbed.
- **The human brain is 60% fat:** Your brain is the fattiest organ in your body. Fat is vital for the proper functioning of the brain.
- **You use the whole of your brain, not only 10% of it:** Every element in your brain is always active.
- **The full development of your brain takes many years, up until you reach 25 years of age:** The growth of the brain does not take place all at once. Actually, your brain develops from the back and continues to the front. Interestingly, the frontal lobes, which are responsible for regulating reasoning and planning are the last to develop.
- **Your brain can generate approximately 23 Watts of power:** This amount of power is

enough to light up a bulb. The power of the brain is maintained by attaining enough exercise and sleep.

The brain is a complex organ that requires proper care for it to function well. It can be a memory reservoir but it can also be prone to forgetting. Damages to the brain can interfere with the organ's functioning ability. Natural aging can also affect the cognitive functions of the brain. In the next chapter, we will delve deeper into the nitty-gritty of cognitive decline and strategies for self-assessing your brain.

2

HOW SHARP ARE YOU?

In every nine adults, one of them has subjective cognitive decline (SCD) (Centers for Diseases Prevention and Control (CDC), 2019). More research has shown that SCD is more prevalent in older people. Statistics revealed that about 11.7% of the people who are aged 65 years and above are prone to experiencing SCD. On the other hand, 10.8% of those who are aged between 45 and 64 also suffer from SCD (CDC, 2019). These numbers show that cognitive decline is an issue of concern among senior citizens. The focus of this chapter hinges upon exploring cognitive decline. We will also look at methods for assessing yourself so that you can determine "how sharp you are."

YOUR BRAIN CHANGES AS YOU AGE

In the same way that other parts of your body might change as you grow, the same happens with your brain. Even your skin loses its elasticity with time, doesn't it? In much the same manner, the cognitive abilities and memory of your brain decline as you age. Let's explore more about these changes in this section.

Cognitive Changes

Some brain functions such as recalling the names of people you have met before tend to take longer as years go by. You might increasingly find it difficult to create new memories about people, events, and tasks. There are three forms of memory that we will describe in association with cognitive changes of the brain and these are:

- **Declarative memory:** This refers to the memory that is associated with information that you would have learned. Remembering life events also fall under this category. This type of memory usually reduces as you grow older.
- **Procedural memory:** This form of memory involves recalling procedures for doing things, from the simplest to the most complex and it remains intact as you age. You can still

remember how to drive a car or tie your grandchildren's shoes, despite their age.

- **Working memory:** This type of memory also tends to decline with age. Working memory involves your ability to keep a piece of information in mind. This could be the location where you parked your car or an old friend's phone number.

Structural Changes

Your brain also undergoes changes in structure and chemistry as time progresses. The changes that take place in your brain as you approach midlife can be successfully measured. As you approach your '40s, your brain begins to significantly shrink. The rate at which your brain shrinks continues to increase as you age, becoming even faster during your '60s. Another point to note is that the shrinking does not take place at a constant rate in all parts of the brain. There are some parts that shrink a bit slower than the others. The hippocampus, prefrontal cortex, and cerebellum shrink at a much faster rate. The loss in these parts of the brain increases as you grow older. The cerebral cortex, which contains cell bodies, thins with increasing age.

Chemical Changes

For your brain to transmit information, you need chemical messengers. Aging usually takes a toll on the production of these chemical messengers so that they are released at a much slower rate. Research has shown that less dopamine is produced by older brains (Wnuk, 2019). In another study, results revealed lower serotonin levels in participants who were 60 and 70 years old (Nichols, 2020).

Neuronal Changes

The structural changes that are noticed in parts of the brain are usually due to the transformation of individual neurons. These neurons shrink as they retract their dendrites. Changes in the neuron structure accompany the deterioration of the fatty myelin that covers the axons of the brain neurons. The connections between your brain cells are also negatively affected as evidenced by their reduction in numbers. The reduced synapses between brain cells cut down on your memory and learning acumen. It is believed that the effects of synaptic changes on cognitive decline are larger and more defined than those that are caused by structural and chemical changes.

As you age, the dendritic spines of neurons become thinner. The dendrites are also altered. The process of neurogenesis, which involves the formation of new neurons, declines. There are two areas of the brain that continue to create new neurons even after birth and these are the dentate gyrus and olfactory bulbs, both of which are found in the hippocampus. The functions of these parts are affected by aging.

MILD COGNITIVE IMPAIRMENT

Mild cognitive impairment (MCI) occurs when an individual shows symptoms of cognitive decline but has not reached the average age for such impairment. However, these symptoms are so mild that they do not interfere with a person's lifestyle. Individuals can still go on with their normal daily routines as usual. In most cases, five years down the line these individuals will be diagnosed with dementia or Alzheimer's disease. It is important to note that MCI is very important in identifying conditions like dementia.

Symptoms of MCI

MCI affects one's ability to decide, think, talk, and remember things. If you have MCI, you will find yourself forgetting some of the most basic things. Some of the most common symptoms of mild cognitive impairment are as follows:

- Being forgetful.
- Finding it difficult to concentrate.
- Finding it difficult to come up with words to finish simple conversations.
- Forgetting important life events.
- Difficulty in making simple decisions.
- Difficulty in analyzing situations or coming up with sound solutions.
- Quickly becoming anxious or irritated.
- Obsessing over minor issues.
- Being depressed or feeling anxious.
- Getting lost.
- Forgetting your password.

Causes of MCI

There are many factors that contribute to MCI. Please note that the symptoms of MCI may also lead to many conditions. Some of the risk factors of MCI are old age, smoking, insomnia, being overweight, as well as having APOE e3, a gene that is associated with Alzheimer's disease. Here is a list of some of the other causes of MCI:

- Shrinking of the part of the brain responsible for memory, which is the hippocampus
- Heart disease
- Diabetes

- Alzheimer's disease
- Parkinson's disease
- Kidney problems
- Shortage of glucose in areas that are important for the brain
- Reduced blood flow in important brain regions
- Strokes
- Lack of exercise
- Brain trauma
- Drug or alcohol abuse

As you get older, your body is most likely not going to be able to function as it used to when you were younger. Your metabolism slows down, making it difficult for your immune system to be able to fight certain illnesses. Performing certain activities becomes a challenge. You become vulnerable to various diseases and this only speeds up your risk of cognitive impairment. In older individuals, cognitive impairment may be caused by any of the following issues:

- After effects of certain medicine
- Hormonal imbalances
- Low metabolism
- Delirium
- Infection
- Malnutrition

- Psychiatric issues

Preventing MCI

As the saying goes, "Prevention is better than cure." There are a number of ways through which you can prevent MCI. Introducing yourself to games that require you to be mentally proactive, like puzzles, may help. Make sure you are staying healthy, especially if you have chronic medical conditions such as heart or kidney failure to avoid their progression. Avoid drug and alcohol abuse, as well as polluted air. We will explore even more preventative measures in this section.

▷ Eat Healthy

Eating healthy is the solution to many health conditions people are facing nowadays. It has become common knowledge that we are what we eat, meaning that if we ingest positive food types, we will recognize better health. Cognitive impairment can be reduced by consuming food that contains B vitamins, antioxidants, fatty acids, and even caffeine. Additionally, Mediterranean dietary habits and eating plans that attempt to lower hypertension are useful in lowering the risk of cognitive decline. Homocysteine is the protein that is responsible for the increase in cognitive impairment. B vitamins help by ensuring that this protein is synthesized. We can get B vitamins from food that are high in protein, and these include beans, meat, and eggs.

Fatty acids, especially omega-3 and omega-6 are important in lowering the risk of cognitive decline. They assist in the formation of supporting structures of neurons. We can get fatty acids from vegetables, fish, or different kinds of nuts. The brain naturally has very low levels of antioxidants. This makes it more susceptible to injury by these oxidative free radicals. An increase in antioxidant intake will ensure that your brain is protected and less likely to experience cognitive impairment. Common examples of antioxidants are vitamin C and A, and they are mainly found in fruits and vegetables.

The Mediterranean dietary habits involve the consumption of food that contains the essential nutrients that are required by the brain. This helps to improve your brain health, thereby lowering the risk of cognitive decline. Eating plans that attempt to lower hypertension are as effective as Mediterranean diets.

▷ **Regular Exercise**

It's no secret that exercise is beneficial to your overall health. Regular exercise has the positive effect of increased blood flow throughout your body, including your brain. Metabolism is constantly occurring in the brain. This process requires an effective transportation system in the brain to ensure that the much needed nutrients are transported to where they need to be. This, in turn, improves your brain's performance. One of the most important functions of your brain is storing memories. Your memory improves through the continuous formation of synapses. Exercising aids this continuous synaptic formation, thereby improving your brain health.

Stress is one of the leading causes of cognitive impairment. This means that a reduction in stress lowers your chances of having to deal with cognitive impairment. Exercise works by reducing the impact of stress on one's brain. This means that the mechanisms that detect stress in the brain are lowered. Hormones called endorphins are released in your body after a workout. These hormones have the ability to make you happy, leading to a reduction in symptoms of stress and anxiety. Exercise improves your health if you are battling with conditions like diabetes and heart disease. These conditions are linked with the development of cognitive impairment. Fighting against such conditions helps you to conquer cognitive impairment.

▷ **Continue Learning New Things**

Just like all the other cells in your body, brain cells keep regenerating. This regeneration of new cells in the brain can be accelerated by exercising your brain. In brief, continuous learning of new things is a strategy for getting your brain to exercise. Keeping your brain active by learning new things can lead to more synapses forming in your brain. There are many ways of learning new things. Playing games like crosswords or puzzles challenges your brain, thereby keeping it active. Such games force you to be conscious and focused on finding the solutions. They require you to use your memory and visual skills, which is just the exercise your brain needs.

You can even decide to go back to school. Academic or practical education will engage your brain more than anything else. Being literate lowers your chances of cognitive impairment. You can try learning new languages or join a book club. This allows you to use your memory as much as possible, improving it. Learning new things gives you the opportunity to learn skills that might actually improve your lifestyle.

▷ Get Enough Sleep

A lot of the activities we are able to perform are activated by our brains and so getting quality sleep is essential. Insomnia or sleep deprivation is one of the leading causes of cognitive impairment (Ebert et al., 2019). When your body is at rest, your brain becomes less active and this allows it to relax.

Sleep has many positive benefits for the brain. It improves your level of attention, your situation analysis skills, and most importantly, it enables your brain to store more information. Sleep occurs in different stages and each stage is accompanied by the excretion of different chemicals in the brain. Depriving your brain of these chemicals will lead to poor brain health. Just like you need a break from your job, your neurons need a break too. If you are not getting quality sleep, then you are overworking your neurons thus increasing your chances of cognitive impairment. Be careful not to sleep for too long, as this might have detrimental effects on your brain, too.

▷ Interact With Others

It is common for people as they get older to start lacking interest in socialization, resulting in fewer friends. The older we get, we witness our friends passing away, moving to other locations, or becoming more involved with grandchildren. However, socializing with others is an essential need for everyone. There is a direct link between having a healthy brain and having a very active social life. Most teenagers have healthy brains because their social life is at its peak. Socializing leads to the creation of many memories that force your brain to pick up its pace in memory storage. Socializing makes you happy, thereby reducing your stress levels. This only leads to great brain health.

Interacting with others can motivate you to step out of your comfort zone and start being active. Joining a Legion or other organization intended for older clients can help introduce you to new activities. Being around people will help you to improve on skills like listening, problem-solving, and concentration. You can also learn some things from your social groups. For example, you can learn a new language or get introduced to a new hobby. All these factors will positively impact your brain.

SELF-ASSESSMENT: ARE YOU AT RISK?

Cognitive impairment is usually accompanied by many signs and symptoms. These symptoms affect speech, sight, and memory. The symptoms that are associated with cognitive impairment may disrupt your ability to maintain your normal daily activities. These symptoms are closely associated with conditions like Alzheimer's disease and dementia. Below is a quiz with nine questions that will attempt to assist you to find out if you have symptoms of dementia. The questions focus on key areas that include concentration, analyzing situations, solution finding, socialization, and different types of memory. It looks at how you use these aspects each day. **Please note**: This is not a diagnostic tool, so it is best to seek help from a health professional before concluding that you have or don't have dementia.

Please note that the last two questions require "yes" or "no" responses. The first seven questions will need you to select one answer among the following options:

- Always
- Never
- Sometimes

1. Is it difficult for you to decide on basic things like your outfit or what to have for breakfast?
2. Do you find it difficult to pay attention while watching a movie or playing a game on your cell phone?
3. Do you use phrases that generalize things because you would have forgotten their names, even things you use almost on a daily basis?
4. Do you forget how to use certain things even though you use them a lot or get lost in places you've been a lot of times?
5. Do you have trouble understanding what other people understand easily? Is it difficult for you to get where the conversation is headed, or find

    yourself saying things that are often viewed as inappropriate by others?

6. Have you had people telling statements like "You've told me that before," or forget appointments or important life events?

7. Do you need assistance when it comes to things like putting on your outfit, what food to eat, sticking to your prescription, or how you use your money?

8. Are these symptoms worsening and becoming more difficult to deal with?

9. Is your life becoming more difficult due to these symptoms, and looking back, do you notice the changes in your capability to handle certain things and situations?

In a nutshell, this chapter has attempted to educate you on subjective cognitive decline. The content explained why MCI is called subjective and how difficult it is to deal with. You've learned about how your brain changes with age and factors that accompany the process. You were introduced to declarative, procedural, and working memory and how each is different and important.

The symptoms that come with mild cognitive impairment (MCI) were also identified. Factors that cause mild cognitive impairment were mentioned. You were also made aware of items that negatively impact the brain and encouraged to stick with the healthy choices. The preventative measures of mild cognitive impairment were reviewed. In the next chapter, we will further explore the benefits of "eating smart."

3

EAT SMART

There is a common saying which says, "You are what you eat." This is a true statement because different kinds of food have various nutrients that they provide to the body and brain. Even more so to the brain. Some food and nutrient sources have been seen to assist in keeping the brain healthy so that your body can be effectively powered. Your brain is the organ that consumes the most energy when compared to the other organs. This chapter will provide in-depth knowledge about the key nutrients and foods to consume when it comes to boosting your brain. Several diets and other lifestyles that you could adopt to help boost your brain health are also included.

IMPORTANT NUTRIENTS

There is a need to fuel your body with healthy food so that the necessary vitamins and nutrients are channeled to your brain. Upon reaching the brain, these nutrients and vitamins help in building the structure, maintain cells in a good working condition, assist in completing tasks, and help you to learn. Some of the major nutrients and vitamins that are important when it comes to brain function are vitamin E, omega-3 fatty acids, antioxidants, choline, and B vitamins. Let's discuss some of these important nutrients and vitamins.

Vitamin E

It is important to note that there are some processes that naturally occur in your body. Some of these processes are helpful whereas others are detrimental to your body. Vitamin E is needed by the brain so that its cells can be protected from damage by the body's natural processes. Inadequate consumption of vitamin E can cause poor coordination, unsteadiness, muscle weakness, and sensory nerve damage.

Omega-3 Fatty Acids

Fatty acids are useful in creating the structure of cells. They are also important in allowing your nervous system to function in a proper manner. In young children, omega-3 fatty acids are essential for their developing brains. Insufficient essential fatty acids in children can result in long-term adverse effects on their brains. In addition to that, children may also face great difficulty in learning when they lack omega-3 fatty acids.

Antioxidants

Some vegetables and fruits such as lettuce, kale, and grapes are good sources of antioxidants. These antioxidants are helpful in the protection of brain cells from damage. It has also been noted that antioxidants are helpful in preventing inflammation and memory loss.

Choline

Another essential nutrient that can be obtained from food is choline. This nutrient is capable of the creation of brain cells and the protection of your nerves. The lack of choline can result in memory dysfunction.

B Vitamins

Vitamins such as B12 and folic acid are essential for making chemicals in the brain. B vitamins are also helpful for breaking down food into components that the brain is able to utilize. These B vitamins are very important to the extent that their lack may result in depression, forgetfulness, low energy, and nerve damage. Some additional effects that are caused by not consuming sufficient B vitamins include having difficulties in learning and thinking.

WHICH FOOD SOURCES PROMOTE GOOD BRAIN HEALTH?

The above-mentioned nutrients can be obtained from different food sources. Some of them include seafood, fish, whole grains, avocadoes, blueberries, and flax and chia seeds. Let's discuss more about these food types in this section.

Seafood and Fish

Fatty fish such as salmon is a rich source of omega-3 fatty acids and are therefore great food for the brain. The healthy fats that are in fatty fish can reduce your risk of heart disease and subsequently also lower your chance of developing a brain disease. Some people may prefer to take fish oil supplements, but however, the best way to obtain your omegas is through the consumption of food. Apart from salmon, you can also add herring, sardines, mackerel, and trout to your diet.

Whole Grains

Whole grains are an awesome source of energy for both your body and brain. In addition to being an energy provider, they also contain numerous vitamins and fiber. They can assist in the protection against heart disease and other health challenges. The types of whole grains to include in your diet are oats, brown rice, bulgur, wild rice, spelled, and quinoa.

Avocados

You can have your avocado on a sandwich, salad, or even on its own. These fruits are loaded with folate, and vitamins C. Furthermore, you can also get omega-3 fatty acids and other healthy fats when you consume avocados.

Blueberries

Blueberries possess numerous antioxidants and flavonoids. These plant chemicals have been seen to be helpful with memory and inflammation as well. Consider adding these fruits to your diet.

Flax and Chia Seeds

You could consider having nuts and seeds as your source of omega-3 fatty acids. Flax and chia seeds are rich in vitamin E. You could also add pistachios, almonds, and walnuts to your diet in order to boost your brain. Pumpkin seeds are also worth considering when it comes to brain health. They are high in antioxidants which help protect your body and brain from damage caused by free radicals. Pumpkin seeds are also rich in zinc, copper, and magnesium. Zinc encourages nerve signaling, copper controls nerve signals, and magnesium is crucial for memory and learning. Iron is another component of pumpkin seeds and is important for the good functioning of the brain.

Coffee

You are on the right track in relation to brain health if you start your mornings with a cup of coffee. The main components of coffee are antioxidants and caffeine, which are great in supporting brain health. Caffeine provides your brain with enhanced alertness, increased concentration, and an improved mood.

Caffeine enhances your brain's alertness by blocking the action of adenosine. This chemical messenger is responsible for making you feel sleepy. According to a certain study, the consumption of caffeine was seen to improve alertness and attention in people who had to complete a cognition test (Jennings, 2021). Another one of caffeine's functions is to boost dopamine, which is one of your neurotransmitters that improves mood. Long-term consumption of coffee has been linked to a lowered risk of Alzheimer's and Parkinson's diseases.

Turmeric

The active ingredient in turmeric is called curcumin and has been mentioned to have numerous benefits for your brain. Curcumin has an intriguing way of functioning because it has the ability to cross the blood-brain barrier. This means that curcumin can directly get into the brain and offer its benefits right away. Curcumin is an anti-inflammatory and antioxidant compound, with benefits that include enhancement of memory, promotion of growth of new brain cells, and easing depression.

Oranges

You can get sufficient vitamin C for a day by eating a medium orange. The vitamin C that you can obtain from consuming an orange is key in preventing mental deterioration. Increased levels of vitamin C are linked with enhanced performance in relation to carrying out tasks that involve memory, attention, decision, speed, and focus. Vitamin C is a strong antioxidant that can combat free radicals that can potentially damage your brain cells. Enhanced brain health, through vitamin C, helps to provide protection against schizophrenia, Alzheimer's disease, anxiety, and major depressive disorder.

Green Tea

Did you know that green tea contains caffeine? The caffeine in green tea brings about its ability to enhance memory, focus, performance, and alertness. Green tea also contains an amino acid called L-theanine that can cross the blood-brain barrier and therefore enhance the activity of the neurotransmitter gamma-aminobutyric acid (GABA). This tends to lower your anxiety and helps in making you feel more relaxed. Green tea is also a good source of polyphenols and antioxidants that help in protecting you from mental decline.

Eggs

Several nutrients are found in eggs such as choline, folate, and vitamins B6 and B12. Choline is used by your body to produce acetylcholine, which is a neurotransmitter that assists in the regulation of memory and mood. The recommended daily intake of choline is 425 mg for women while that of men is 550 mg (Jennings, 2021). Bear in mind that a single egg yolk contains 112 mg of choline. The B vitamins that are found in eggs help to lessen the effects of Alzheimer's disease and dementia. Having enough folate and the B vitamins can help to counteract depression. Consuming adequate folate helps in the reduction of age-related mental deterioration. The other functions of vitamin

B12 are to control sugar levels in the brain and to synthesize brain chemicals.

Broccoli

Broccoli is rich in vitamin K and antioxidants. The vitamin K in this vegetable is very high such that one cup of cooked broccoli is able to deliver more than 100% of the Recommended Daily Intake. Vitamin K intake is largely associated with enhanced cognitive status and memory. In addition to the antioxidant properties, broccoli also has anti-inflammatory properties that can assist in the protection against brain damage.

Dark Chocolate

Dark chocolate contains antioxidants, caffeine, and flavonoids, all of which are important for boosting your brain. Flavonoids are mainly linked with learning and memory. According to research, flavonoids assist in slowing down age-related mental deterioration and improves memory (Jennings, 2021). Chocolate is also popularly known as a mood booster.

Fermented Foods

Fermented foods are also an option in relation to foods that promote good brain health. Research revealed that consuming six servings of fermented foods can reduce inflammation (Parker-Pope, 2022). Fermented foods include sauerkraut, yogurt, kefir, kombucha, and kimchi.

Leafy Greens

Leafy greens such as kale, spinach, arugula, and beet greens are good sources of vitamins C and A, folate, and fiber. Apart from salads, you can add your greens to stews, soups, smoothies, or stir-fries. Consider helping yourself to servings of leafy greens for the improvement of your brain health.

BEST DIETS FOR A BETTER BRAIN

It is noteworthy that, for you to improve brain functions, a combination of diets should be employed. In addition to diets, adopting certain habits may also work to your advantage in terms of enhancing your brain cells. Some of the important diets that you can employ include the Dietary Approaches to Stop Hypertension (DASH), Mediterranean, and the Mediterranean-DASH Intervention for Neurodegenerative Delay (MIND). When looking at the components of each of them, these three diets are similar (WebMD Editorial Contributors, 2021). Some of the important habits that you could adopt include having a low consumption of processed foods, sugar, and alcohol.

Dietary Approaches to Stop Hypertension (DASH)

The DASH diet comprises foods that are rich in magnesium, calcium, and potassium while limiting foods that have high amounts of saturated fats, added sugars, and sodium. Foods that are included in this diet include whole grains, fruits, and vegetables. Low-fat dairy or fat-free products, nuts, beans, fish, and poultry are also components of this diet.

The Mediterranean Diet

The Mediterranean diet consists of staple foods for the people who reside in countries that are around the Mediterranean Sea. These countries include Italy, France, Spain, Croatia, and Greece. The Mediterranean diet is mainly centered on consuming foods that are plant-based. In addition to that, the diet also includes healthy fats such as olive oil and omega-3 fatty acids that are found in fish. Fruits, vegetables, whole grains, legumes, nuts, and seafood are the other constituents of the Mediterranean diet. When you have decided to adopt this diet, you have to completely avoid or limit your intake of red meat, sugary foods, refined grains, and dairy. However, your dairy intake may include small amounts of cheese and yogurt.

It is worth noting that the Mediterranean diet allows you to have low to moderate amounts of red wine.

Moderate, in this case, refers to having a glass of wine on a daily basis (Migala, 2020). Although the Mediterranean diet gives an allowance to take some wine, you should note that it is not an encouragement to start having it if you do not already take it.

Numerous benefits are associated with the consumption of the Mediterranean diet. Some of the benefits include the regulation of blood sugar levels, enhanced heart health, and brain function support. A number of studies have also reported that the Mediterranean diet can assist in the prevention of heart attacks and the promotion of weight loss (Gunnars, 2021). Strokes, premature death, and type 2 diabetes can also be prevented if you are on a Mediterranean diet.

We mentioned earlier that the Mediterranean diet is beneficial for healthy brain cells. As you get older, this diet can also help to protect against cognitive decline. This was shown in a study that included 512 people who strongly adhered to the Mediterranean diet (Gunnars, 2021). Their enhanced memory and lower risk factors for Alzheimer's disease were attributed to their adherence to the diet. The Mediterranean diet has also been linked to reduced risks of cognitive impairment, dementia, and Alzheimer's disease. A review study has also revealed enhanced processing speed, attention, memory, and cognitive function in older adults that had adopted the Mediterranean diet.

Following the Mediterranean Diet

By now, you have a better understanding of the Mediterranean diet, its components, and its advantages as well. If you are interested in following this diet, you have to plan your meals in a certain way. For example, your meals have to be built around whole grains, beans, and vegetables. When you are preparing your food, avoid using butter, and substitute it with olive oil. Also, consider having fish at least two times per week. For your dessert, you should serve fresh fruit.

Mediterranean-DASH Intervention for Neurodegenerative Delay (MIND)

The MIND diet is a combination of the DASH and the Mediterranean diets. This diet is mainly centered on food groups that are found in each of the diets that are responsible for improving your brainpower and at the same time, protecting it from age-based problems such as Alzheimer's disease (Sreenivas, 2021). Basically, the MIND diet allows you to consume a total of up to 10 food groups, and no less than five. In essence, on a daily basis, you should consume at least three servings of whole grains, vegetables, and fruits. In addition to that, you can eat a serving or two of beans, fish, and poultry each week. For your daily snacks, you can include berries and nuts. This diet also strongly encourages you to use olive oil as a fat source that is healthy for cooking your food.

The Mediterranean diet recommends that you sparingly consume meat and dairy products for your meals. You may not entirely cut them out but you could consume them approximately less than four times a week. Instead of having meat and dairy in your diet, you could substitute them with legumes and beans that are more likely to be beneficial for the health of your brain. Here is a list of foods that you should consume when you are on a MIND diet.

- **Olive oil:** Consume this daily, through cooked meals of salad dressing.
- **Berries:** Eat two or more servings per week.
- **Green leafy vegetables:** Examples of leafy greens include spinach, collard greens, and kale. Include at least one serving on a daily basis.
- **All other vegetables:** Eat two or more servings on a daily basis.
- **Whole grains:** Have three or more servings per day.
- **Poultry:** Eat two or more servings per week.
- **Beans:** Consume at least four or more servings per week.

- **Seafood or fish:** Eat one or more servings per week (we recommend fatty fish such as sardines, mackerel, herring, and salmon).

Bear in mind that there are also foods that you have to limit or avoid when you are on the MIND diet. Limiting or avoiding these foods will come in handy when it comes to maintaining your brain in a healthy state. Here is a list of foods that you should avoid or limit:

- Red meat
- Margarine or butter
- Sweets and pastries
- Cheese

Benefits of Following the MIND Diet

By now, you have an idea of what foods to consume on a MIND diet in order to boost your brain health. In addition to the type of foods that you could consume, the recommended amounts are given above. These food groups are beneficial because they include nutrients such as carotenoids, flavonoids, omega-3 fatty acids, folate, and vitamin E.

The MIND diet has been shown to enhance your brain health and reduce your chances of developing dementia, Alzheimer's disease, and other types of age-related cognitive decline. Whether or not you have a family history of these diseases or not, please note that following this diet will come in handy in relation to boosting your brain. In actual fact, numerous studies have revealed that the consumption of certain foods and the shunning of unhealthy ones can cause the reduction of the aging of the brain by a total of 7.5 years (Sreenivas, 2021).

The statistics in the U.S. concerning the occurrence of Alzheimer's show that the disease is sixth in causing death. It is also estimated to have effects on a total of over five million people in America. This is a very high number, considering the fact that there are ways that one could employ to evade this disease. Therefore, it is recommended to adopt the MIND diet in order to counter the effects of Alzheimer's. It is also important to engage your doctor when you want to start on this diet. A licensed dietician or nutritionist may also help you how to get started on this diet. When you engage a professional, they are more likely to assist you in coming up with a meal plan that will work best to your advantage.

OTHER STRATEGIES FOR BETTER BRAIN HEALTH

Please note that apart from diet there are other strategies that you can utilize to boost your brain health. Some of them include reducing your intake of alcohol, taking your medications, and lowering your sugar intake. To add to that you could also consider practicing mindfulness. Let's discuss these strategies and more in this section.

Low Sugar

Low sugar consumption is advantageous to your health. This is because a high consumption can result in sluggishness, tiredness, and brain fog. Please note that having a poor diet that contains excess sugar can cause you to lose essential structures and brain activities. Consuming excess sugar can aggravate dementia and the aging of your brain.

Low Alcohol

It has been noted that drinking alcohol can impact your brain (WebMD Editorial Contributors, 2021). Drinking alcohol can cause you to be more relaxed. However, drinking it in excessive amounts can result in anxiety and depression. Chronic heavy drinking can also result in permanent changes as well as damage to the brain. In

America, it has been noted that approximately 2.6 percent of deaths are caused by alcohol (Villines, 2021).

We mentioned earlier that alcohol can change the chemistry of the brain. If you consume alcohol, the activity of Gamma-aminobutyric acid (GABA) is increased. GABA is the primary inhibitory neurotransmitter that is found in the brain. When in high amounts, it causes the suppression of neuron activity thereby resulting in slowed reflexes, lapses in short-term memory, unsteady gait, and slurred speech. The changes in brain chemistry that occur after someone has consumed alcohol may cause them to experience a number of moods such as confusion, aggression, anger, mania, and euphoria. Please note that if a person has had too much to drink in a short space of time, they may experience a slow breathing and heart rate, thereby resulting in a coma.

In the long term, heavy drinking can cause structural abnormalities or chronic changes in the activity of the neurotransmitters. A number of adverse effects have been noted that result from the abuse of alcohol. Among the effects are cardiovascular health issues, dementia, poor circulation to the brain, and brain shrinkage. Furthermore, you may also be exposed to nutritional deficiencies that injure the brain or lead to an alcohol-based type of dementia known as Korsakoff syndrome.

Other negative effects that result from the long-term abuse of alcohol include changes in personality or mood and the development of mental health issues such as psychosis and hallucinations. If exposed to alcohol, babies and children experience stunted brain development. It is important for pregnant women to stay away from alcohol. If you take alcohol during pregnancy, your unborn baby may develop an intricate group of symptoms that are referred to as fetal alcohol syndrome.

It is now clear to you just how drinking alcohol can cause negative effects on your body, especially the brain. You may have had a drinking problem for a long time, but it is important to consider quitting. By eliminating alcohol, some adverse alcohol-related brain damage and premature death can be prevented. Furthermore, the risk of continued brain damage can be reduced if you quit drinking alcohol. In cases where you are facing difficulties trying to stop drinking, organizations such as the highly effective Alcoholics Anonymous (AA) can assist, or consider independent mental health support. You could also avoid places or people that may influence you to drink.

Take Your Medications

It is possible that you may be suffering from a certain disease. This disease may be a mental health ailment or it can be any other condition such as a thyroid one, which is capable of affecting your brain. In this case, ensure that you keep your brain healthy by religiously taking your medications as directed by your physician.

Remain Active

Numerous advantages are associated with exercise as we highlighted earlier. When you exercise, you tend to keep a healthy weight. This is advantageous in that your risk of developing heart disease is reduced. Subsequently, brain chemicals that assist in the improvement of your mood are then produced. It is, therefore, crucial to remain active so that you stay healthy.

Consider Practicing Mindfulness

Mindfulness encourages you to focus on the moment and think things through before doing them in a haphazard and unproductive manner. Eliminating distractions and extraneous thoughts allows your brain to focus on the task at hand, reducing stress. Your brain is put to good use and you are more likely to produce remarkable outcomes when you practice mindfulness. Furthermore, if you learn to be in the present moment, you tend to be calm and more focused. As a result, you are in a better position to have a sense of well-being and enhanced mental health.

Quit Smoking

For some, smoking may be an activity that they do in order to relieve stress. However, there are a lot of adverse effects that result from this activity. Some of the common effects of smoking are the development of cancer, strokes, and heart disease. These ailments will negatively affect your brain, therefore, it is advisable for you to quit smoking.

In Chapter 3, we discussed some of the negative actions we take that can cause our brain to deteriorate. Next, we will focus on an area that has a positive influence on brain health: exercise and movement.

4

MOVE TO NOT LOSE YOUR MIND

Exercise is really for the brain, not the body. It affects mood, vitality, alertness, and feeling of well-being.

— JOHN RATEY

Regular exercise plays an important role in living a good healthy lifestyle. Movement or exercise is a key component of improving your brain and preventing cognitive impairment. Exercise is not only good for your muscles and bones, but it also plays an important role in keeping your brain healthy. It improves your short and long-term memory. The more you exercise, the more you remember a lot of things you did and the things you are supposed to do. Constantly working out keeps your mind very sharp.

Consistent exercise does not mean only playing sports. Anything that will keep your body active and moving will do. If you are not good at playing sports, do not worry, you can do other exercises such as swimming, biking, dancing, and walking, just to mention a few. I use long walks, jogging, and/or dancing to relieve stress and keep moving.

During exercise, your body releases dopamine and endorphins, which makes you feel happy. Exercising reduces stress and boosts your mood. When you are upset, completing some form of exercise can help to control and reset your emotions. This chapter focuses on exercise and your brain health. The benefits of exercising, how exercise boosts your brain health, and why it is recommended to move so as not to lose your mind will be discussed in detail.

EXERCISE AND BRAIN HEALTH

Regular exercise increases your muscle size and reduces the amount of fat in your body. It changes the shape of your body tissues. When you exercise, you will be changing the structure of your brain as well. It helps you to protect your memory as you age. Exercise has the ability to reduce insulin resistance, stimulate the release of growth factors, and reduce inflammation. The growth factors are the chemicals that affect the growth of brain cells, new blood vessels in the brain, and survival of new brain cells.

Exercising helps you to concentrate, feel mentally sharp, and reduce the effects of stress. Endorphins play an important role in making you feel better. Exercise helps you to improve your sleep, in addition to dealing with anxiety, depression, and more. This section will shed some light on why and how exercise protects your brain's health.

How Does Exercise Help the Brain?

Regular exercise helps your brain in several ways. It stimulates the release of body hormones that are involved in the growth of brain cells. Exercise increases your heart rate, so oxygen is made more available to your brain. It increases your mental abilities as mentioned earlier. If you are active during the day, it means you will sleep better at night.

The protein called the brain neurotrophic factor (BDNF) is triggered by exercise. This protein encourages the growth of new brain cells. You should boost your BDNF through exercise so that you reduce the risk of schizophrenia, anxiety, and depression. Brain-derived neurotrophic factor promotes the occurrence of changes in your brain. Exercise reduces inflammation, contributes to neural growth, and enhances the formation of new patterns in brain functions that promote the feeling of well-being and calmness. Endorphins and other powerful chemicals that are released during exercise energize you and you will feel good. Here are other ways through which exercise improves your brain health.

▷ Promoting Cardiovascular Health

Exercising will help you if you want to reduce the risk of cardiovascular diseases. If you reduce the risk of obesity, high blood pressure, and abnormal values of lipids, you will also cut down the possibility of occurrence of cardiac events. Exercising is the best way to decrease risk factors that cause cardiac disease. When you exercise regularly, you are more likely to reduce your body weight, increase insulin sensitivity, and increase exercise tolerance.

▷ Improving Blood Flow to the Brain

Exercise increases the rate at which your blood flows to the brain. As you start to exercise, your heart rate increases and blood flow increases to the brain. When you exercise your brain becomes exposed to more oxygen and nutrients. Beneficial proteins are released to promote growth of neurons in the brain. Release of nutrients require more energy and all the processes occur when there is an increase in heart rate which aids more blood flow to your brain. High energy during exercise requires more blood so the brain and heart work hand-in-hand to fill the need. Your brain uses its muscles to increase reaction time during exercise and produce waste, such as lactic acid. The lactic acid is carried away from the muscles and this is more efficient when the rate of blood flow to the brain is rapid.

When you exercise, your muscles dilate, thus improving your blood flow. ATP is an energy-carrying molecule that stores and distributes energy throughout the whole body. When ATP is used up in your muscles, metabolic products such as hydrogen ions, adenosine, and carbon dioxide are produced. They leave your muscle cells with thin-walled blood vessels so that they dilate. This is called vasodilation. Capillaries increase the flow of blood and this will cause more blood supply to your working muscle.

▷ **Contributes to Neurogenesis**

Your brain continues to produce neurons that control your memory and thinking. This process that is known as neurogenesis occurs to increase your brain volume and this process helps you to buffer against dementia. Exercising triggers neurogenesis, which aids you with greater brain plasticity. Exercising also increases the production of neurotransmitters in your brain. Neurotransmitters help you to boost mood and information processing.

▷ Decreasing Feelings of Anxiety

You should exercise to reduce the sensitivity of your body to anxiety. Regular exercise reduces the occurrence of irritable bowel syndrome which is a common condition. Exercising aids the growth of neurons in your brain. Neurons help in relieving the occurrence of psychiatric conditions including anxiety and depression.

▷ Improving Your Focus and Concentration

Exercise improves your learning and memory acumen. If you do not exercise, you can experience brain fog which is a clouding of consciousness. Symptoms of brain fog are lack of concentration, difficulties in remembering things, and poor focus. Brain fog is caused by fatigue, depression, anxiety, nutritional deficiencies, and hormonal shifts. Exercise decreases brain fog and increases your concentration.

▷ Protecting Your Brain from Aging and Neurodegenerative Diseases

You should exercise to increase your life expectancy. Exercising has neurological benefits, which include a decrease in stress, improved emotion processing, and increased focus. The occurrence of neurodegenerative diseases decreases when you exercise.

THE MENTAL HEALTH BENEFITS OF EXERCISE

Regular exercise is not just for increasing your muscle size and for your aerobic capacity. It also improves your physique, trims your waistline, increases your life expectancy, and physical health, and can increase your sex life. You spend the whole day energetic and sleep well at night due to movement during the day. The more you practice, the more your memory becomes sharp and you tend to feel positive about your life.

Mental and physical energy can be boosted through exercise. When you are stressed, your muscles become tense, most likely in your neck, shoulders, and face, possibly leaving you with a headache. You experience insomnia, diarrhea, frequent urination, heartburn, cramps in your muscles, and stomachache. This will lead to more stress and there will be no proper function and communication between the body and the brain. You can stop this by exercising. As you start to exercise, your muscles relax and the tension in the body is relieved. Your body and your brain work hand in hand and they are linked, if the body relaxes, your mind relaxes too.

Exercise and Attention Deficit Hyperactivity Disorder

Exercising is one of the ways through which you can reduce the symptoms of Attention Deficit Hyperactivity Disorder (ADHD). Regular activity boosts your brain's norepinephrine, dopamine, and serotonin levels. These affect your focus and concentration. In this way, exercise works the same as the ADHD medications, such as Adderall and Ritalin. Exercising helps you to relax when you have ADHD. Exercising provides your body with more energy, helps to motivate your mental tasks, and boosts your brain power.

You should consider your exercise as a treatment dose. We recommend that you exercise for at least thirty minutes a day. Depending on the type of sport or exercise program, make sure you are maintaining at least a moderately intense level. With ADHD, you should do aerobic exercises. You should make sure that you sweat during the activity, that your muscles feel tired, you breathe harder and fast, and your heart rate increases. If you are not sure about how intense your exercise should be, consult your doctor.

With aerobic exercises, you create new pathways in the brain, which will increase the way you pay attention. For you to raise your heart rate, you should run, walk briskly, and do biking. For a start, if you are not able to run fast, you should start by jogging. Also consider doing other exercises such as push-ups, lunges, and weightlifting.

Exercise Against Post Traumatic Stress Disorder and Trauma

Post-traumatic stress disorder (PTSD) is a mental disorder that develops when you are exposed to a traumatic scenario, such as a natural disaster, serious accident, war, terrorist attack, or personal assault like rape or home invasion. Post-traumatic stress disorder affects your feelings and thoughts, and causes physical distress. Survivors of trauma develop anxiety, depression, and mood disorder.

Symptoms of PTSD include panic and hyper-vigilance, including angry outbursts. If you are exercising with PTSD, your heart beats very fast, your blood pressure increases, and this can lead to shortness of breath. You should workout because exercising provides lubrication in the whole body and will help you to reduce the trauma effect, depression, and anxiety. Limited movement is best if you have PTSD. This will help you to maintain the recommended breathing rate.

Sharpens Your Memory and Way of Thinking

Exercise sharpens your memory and thinking. Endorphins help you to increase concentration and your reasoning capacity. Regular exercise sharpens your brain and makes you feel mentally aware. It aids in the growth of new brain cells and your life expectancy.

Higher Self-Esteem

Exercising boosts mood, which inturn helps you feel a sense of achievement in your life. When you workout, you start to feel better about your body and appearance when you are with others. It makes you feel more powerful. If you set certain goals or exercise targets and meet them, you increase your overall confidence.

Better Sleep, More Energy, and More Resilience

It is best to exercise during the day so that you will sleep well at night. You should exercise to let the muscles stretch so that you will relax at night. You gain more energy by doing workouts and the body gets used to using more energy. When you face mental challenges, exercising will help to build resilience and respond to the situation in a healthier way. Exercising boosts your immune system.

EXERCISE AND LET YOUR BRAIN BENEFIT

Exercise helps your brain in different ways as mentioned earlier. Here are some of the ways how exercise helps your brain.

- **Reaping the mental health benefits of exercise is easier than you think:** It is very easy to start exercising and it does not need too much effort. Once you start exercising, you will discover that it will become your hobby. You should start by giving yourself a certain time you consider to be for exercising purposes. For example, if you want to exercise by running, it is better for you to start by walking, jogging and finally, you will be able to run for longer periods.

- **Even a little bit of exercise is better than nothing:** Prioritizing even a small amount of exercise three times per week can start you on your way to a routine. You can start by setting a target at a specific time. You should sit for at least twenty minutes of exercising for the first time. As you continue exercising, you increase the time and increase the intensity of the exercises. As you continue exercising, you will see the benefits of exercising.

- **You don't have to suffer to get results:** You should exercise to be strong physically and mentally. Don't over-exercise or aim for an extravagant goal on the first day. Start small and improve as you go.

OVERCOMING OBSTACLES TO EXERCISE

Exercising makes you feel better but you may face obstacles before or after exercising. You can come across these challenges, especially when you already have some mental health issues. Some of the obstacles that hinder exercising include:

- **Feeling hopeless:** As we mentioned earlier, exercising is very easy. You should be taking light exercise so that you boost your muscle and increase your energy. As you continue exercising, you expand your exercising skills and start to demand more. At first, you might experience loss of hope but it's normal, you should take it easy and start slow. You can even start by making exercising more fun through activities like dancing.

- **Feeling bad about yourself:** You should always think positively about your body. Do not criticize yourself. Do not consider your age, weight, height, or fitness. Just exercise, there are plenty of other people like you. You can consider asking your colleague or sibling to exercise with you. Even if you accomplish the smallest fitness goals, this will help you to gain confidence day and the way you think about yourself.

- **Feeling pain:** Exercising can come with some pain, especially if you are just starting. This can hinder you from continuing with the workout activities. Try to ignore the pain and concentrate on exercising. Your muscles will get used to exercising as time goes on. You can experience joint discomfort, but to decrease that, you should downsize your activities or decrease the time you take when exercising. You should consult your doctor on how safely you can take your exercises.

STARTING YOUR EXERCISES AGAINST A MENTAL HEALTH ISSUE

When you are feeling depressed, stressed, or feeling anxious, the best way to go about it is to exercise. Exercise always makes you feel better. In this section, we will explore strategies that can make you win at making working out a habit.

Start Small

You should start exercising to meet small goals for you to enjoy exercising. You can start by considering 20 minutes per day for your activity. Five times per week is enough for you when you are exercising and having a mental issue. It depends on how likely you are going to follow through your exercises. If your exercises are too ambitious, probably you can feel bad about them and you give up. It is better for you to start with easy exercises so that you can archive them. You will build confidence through small and easy exercises leading you to move to challenging goals. We encourage you to start with small exercises and move on as you meet your goals you will start to demand challenging goals.

Schedule Workouts When Your Energy is Highest

When you feel that you have got a lot of energy, you should do something that drains your energy. You should do the activity you like the most. Activities you enjoy will leave you with a sense of accomplishment and purpose and will let you use the whole of your energy. If you enjoy gardening, window shopping or any other activities, go for them. Performing such activities will help you relax if you are in a negative mood.

Be Comfortable and Reward Yourself

When you exercise, you should put on clothes that you feel comfortable with depending on the type of exercise you are taking. You should reward yourself after every exercise. This will motivate you to continue exercising. You can reward yourself with a favorite episode you like to watch on your TV, for example.

Before you do your favorite activity as a reward, it is important that you tell yourself, "This is my reward for training today." You can either think about it actively or say it loud to yourself. This means that you rely on internal rewards and not as much on external rewards. Outcomes from other people and the environment outside you are what we are referring to as external rewards. Internal rewards are outcomes that result from the actual performance of the task, which in this case, is exercising. The internal rewards will give you a sense of achievement and personal worth.

Make Exercise a Social Activity

You should exercise with your loved ones so that you enjoy exercising. For example, you can exercise with your partner, sibling, or kids. Exercising becomes enjoyable and fun when you make it a social activity. When you are suffering from depression or stress it will become easier to share with your loved ones during the activity.

EASY WAYS TO MOVE MORE THAT DON'T INVOLVE THE GYM

Exercising does not necessarily mean you have to go to the gym. It includes any type of activity which is movement. You should move in and in and around your apartment. You can clean your house, wash your car, mow your lawn, or sweep your room. All these are activities that are not related to the gym. Even without the gym, you can do it.

You should sneak activities that help you to exercise. For example, you can decide to take up stairs instead of elevators. You should walk vigorously instead of drinking coffee during your coffee break. You can do body weight exercises. Body weight exercises burn your calories, improves your body balance, and strengthens your body. There is no need for gym equipment when you are doing this. You can do wall sits. This way of exercising does not involve movement. Wall sits can sound like a boring exercise but it involves a lot of muscle groups and causes burning of extra calories. If you need your body to leverage, you should do wall sits.

Boxing is another excellent way of exercise you can practice and can train your mind as well. You can do boxing for beginners to work out while you are at home. You can do this using your body weight. If you want to warm up, do a rope less classic jump rope. Dancing is another way of exercising without going to the gym. Dancing does not only make you happy but it also tones your entire body. You should turn on your favorite music and start dancing so that you will gain physical fitness.

MAKE EXERCISE A FUN PART OF, YOUR EVERYDAY LIFE

Exercising should be part of your everyday life. This is very easy to do and here are some tips that can help you to fit in your workouts. You should plan for your workouts. Make a rough draft with a list of the workouts that you want to do. To enjoy your exercises more, you should join a team or a league. Working out with your loved ones, co-workers, or friends will help boost your mood while exercising your brain. Make exercise a part of your regular activities. Practice squats, push-ups, and planks. If you have physical limitations with your joints, consider chair yoga or other modifications. These workouts can be done while watching your favorite channel on your TV.

Getting involved in exercising is one of the factors that contribute to neuroplasticity, which in turn increases brain health. We will explore more on neuroplasticity in the next chapter.

5

THE POWER OF NEUROPLASTICITY, PURPOSE, AND DISCOVERY

Any man could, if he were so inclined, be the sculptor of his own brain.

— SANTIAGO RAMÓN Y CAJAL

Positive physiological changes are experienced through the release of adrenaline when we are concentrating intently. Maintaining the level of focus requires the release of acetylcholine in the brain to mark the material for later retrieval. A good sleep or guided meditation through tools such as Yoga Nidra, are two of the functions that help to enhance neuroplasticity. Understanding the positive benefits of adequate rest, regular exercise, and attentiveness provides the motivation to maintain a healthy brain.

The brain is able to alter its structure so that it becomes better suited to perform the necessary tasks. When you have a certain purpose, your brain tends to function accordingly so that the purpose gets fulfilled. It has been noted that when you have a strong sense of purpose you are more likely to live longer. The mortality rate of people with a low sense of purpose is higher as opposed to those with a high sense of purpose. After reading this chapter you will have a deeper understanding of these and related issues.

NEUROPLASTICITY

Have you ever noticed that depending on what is happening in your life or how you interact with your environment, your brains are able to adapt? This ability for the brain to get accustomed to different situations is referred to as neuroplasticity. Let's discuss these and other related issues in this section.

A Brief History

The Polish neuroscientist, Jerzy Konorski, was the first to use the term "neuroplasticity" in 1948 when he observed neuronal structure changes. Although the term was first used by Konorski, the idea has been noted to date back to the 1900s when the father of neuroscience, Santiago Ramón y Cajal, postulated about neuronal plasticity. Cajal recognized that upon reaching adulthood, their brains could change.

In the 1960s, it was found that neurons were able to "reorganize" after the occurrence of a traumatic event. According to further research, stress was noted to change the structure and functions of the brain. Although not conclusive, researchers, in the 1990s, postulated that brain cells can be destroyed by stress. As time progressed, research suggested the idea of replenishment of the brain (Ackerman, 2018).

Neuroplasticity and Neurogenesis

Neuroplasticity involves the formation of new pathways and connections in the brain whereas neurogenesis is the brain's ability to grow new neurons. When compared, neurogenesis seems to be a better option than neuroplasticity. This is because neurogenesis can actually open up new avenues when it comes to the treatment and prevention of dementia, traumatic brain injuries, or other related ailments.

THE THEORY AND PRINCIPLES OF NEUROPLASTICITY

According to neuroscientists McEachern and Shaw, the definition of neuroplasticity is not mutually agreed upon. They suggest the existence of two main perspectives which state that:

- Neuroplasticity is a process that defines any change in behavioral response or final neural activity, or
- Neuroplasticity is a vast collection of various brain alteration and adaptation phenomena.

These perspectives bring out the fact that there is no unifying theory. However, there are two main types of neuroplasticity, which are structural and functional.

- Structural neuroplasticity refers to a type of neuroplasticity in which changes occur in the strength of neuron connections.
- Functional neuroplasticity refers to the permanent changes that occur in synapses as a result of development and learning.

NEUROPLASTICITY AND PSYCHOLOGY

Another potential avenue that neuroplasticity can offer is the provision of psychological changes. At your disposal, there are already chemicals or medications that you can utilize to alter the way your brain functions. In addition to these chemicals, psychology has provided numerous ways to modify human thought patterns. One such way is through learning.

The Relationship Between Neuroplasticity and Learning

It is important to note that when you learn something, new pathways are formed in your brain. As each new lesson comes, it potentially connects new neurons and alters your brain's old way of operating. Neuroplasticity is dependent on how interested you are in learning and how you generally approach life (Ackerman, 2018).

The Relationship Between Neuroplasticity and Age

You may expect neuroplasticity to change as you age. It is indeed true that neuroplasticity changes with age. However, it is not as black and white as many might think. It is essential to note that there are several factors that are involved.

▷ Neuroplasticity in Children

As children grow, their brains also develop and change. Structural or functional changes may occur due to each experience they encounter. To support the idea that neuroplasticity in children changes as they grow, at birth they will have around 7,500 neuronal connections in each neuron, which will double by the age of two (Ackerman, 2018). The main types of neuroplasticity that can be seen in children include adaptive, impaired, excessive, and plasticity which exposes the brain to injury. These types allow children to quickly recover from injury, if any, as compared to the recovery process in adults.

▷ Neuroplasticity in Adults

Neuroplasticity is most common in children. The phenomenon is lower in adults. However, it is possible for the adult brain to restore old connections and functions that have been idle for some time. Memory can also be enhanced and the overall cognitive skills may be enhanced as well. In adults, neuroplasticity can be improved by factors such as a healthy lifestyle and sustained effort.

RESEARCH AND STUDIES ON NEUROPLASTICITY

Brain health is so interesting that many researchers have decided to explore more about it. Different researchers have decided to look at various aspects of this topic. Let's take time to look at some of the developments that have been occurring lately.

- In 2002, it was noted that if you have ten-hourly sessions of cognitive training over a period of five or six weeks, you can possibly reverse the same amount of age-related deterioration that has been seen in a similar time period.
- In 2002, then 2014, research revealed that neuroplasticity can be promoted by enriched environments. They also suggested that enriched environments are able to provoke positive adaptation and growth even after early childhood and young adulthood.
- A study carried out in 2013 suggested that the same level of maturation has been observed for "newborn" neurons at eight weeks and for those who are older.

- Research on intermittent fasting, in 2014, was seen to promote adaptive responses in synapses.
- According to a study carried out in 2014, enough sleep may improve neurogenesis while chronic insomnia is related to damage and death of neurons in the hippocampus.
- Again in 2014, it was observed that good physical fitness has several benefits including preventing or slowing age-related neuronal death and damage to the hippocampus. Furthermore, the volume of the hippocampus can be increased.

HOW NEUROPLASTICITY FUNCTIONS

In the early years of childhood, there is rapid brain growth, which concurs with the presence of numerous synapses per neuron. However, as you grow into adulthood, the number of synapses declines. This is because, as you gain new experiences, some connections are strengthened whereas others are destroyed. The process is called synaptic pruning. Through the pruning process, the brain develops an ability to adapt to changes in the environment.

BENEFITS OF NEUROPLASTICITY

Neuroplasticity works in an interesting manner as we have just seen in the previous section. There are numerous benefits associated with neuroplasticity. Some of them are listed here:

- It provides you with an opportunity to learn new things.
- It can enhance deteriorated or lost functions.
- Neuroplasticity helps to improve already existing cognitive abilities.
- It provides improvements that can enhance brain fitness.
- Helps to allow recovery from traumatic brain damage and strokes.

FACTORS AFFECTING NEUROPLASTICITY

Neuroplasticity can be affected by a number of factors. Age and the environment have been seen to be one of the drivers. Let's discuss more about this topic in this section.

- **Age and environment are influencers:** Although plasticity can occur throughout life, some changes are more dominant at particular ages. We discussed earlier that young people's brains are more sensitive in comparison with older ones. However, with more practice and living a healthy life, older brains can easily adapt. The brain's plasticity can also be influenced by both the environment and genetic factors.

- **Neuroplasticity is an ongoing process:** Plasticity has been observed to continue throughout life. Apart from neurons, it involves other brain cells such as vascular and glial cells. Neuroplasticity occurs due to memory formation, experience, injury to the brain, or learning. When some parts of the brain are damaged, other parts may take over the functions, thereby restoring the abilities.

- **Brain plasticity possesses some limitations:** Please note that as much as other parts of the brain are able to take over damaged functions, it is difficult to restore some of them. Other parts of the brain play crucial roles such as speech, language, and movement. Once these are damaged, it may be difficult to restore them.

HOW TO REWIRE YOUR BRAIN WITH NEUROPLASTICITY

We discussed that, with neuroplasticity, it is possible to rewire your brain. There are several ways that you could use to rewire your brain. Did you know that by merely traveling, you could rewire your brain? Other people may prefer using mnemonic devices as a way of rewiring. In addition to that, you may prefer to do intermittent fasting, learn a musical instrument, or perform non-dominant hand exercises.

You may get new ideas that can help you to rewire your brain if you read fiction. Expanding your vocabulary is another way to rewire your brain. Some may prefer to do artwork when they think of rewiring their brain. Creating artwork has a certain inherent serenity about it, thereby helping you generate other connections in your brain. Furthermore, dancing or better yet, sleeping can assist in relation to brain rewiring. Consider doing one or more of these activities in order to improve your neuroplasticity.

Protocol for Neuroplasticity Improvement

When it comes to maintaining your aging brain, it is important to improve your neuroplasticity. There are several ways that you could use including being focused, alert, doing repetitions, and not being hard on yourself. Let's discuss these and more in this section.

▷ Be Alert

For you to be able to trigger neuroplasticity, it is important to be alert. To do this, simply do about 25-30 deep breaths. Afterward, exhale and hold your breath, making sure that your lungs are empty for approximately 15-60 seconds. You should then inhale once before holding your breath. Once you feel the urge to breathe, go ahead and do that normally. By practicing alertness like this, epinephrine tends to be released in your brain and body.

▷ Be Focused

Mental focus goes hand-in-hand with visual focus. Stare at a point on a screen or wall for about 30-60 seconds to enhance your focus on a particular task. It is normal, though, to experience some disturbances in your focus. Note that this exercise can help in the release of acetylcholine and other mechanisms are activated as well.

▷ Consider Doing Repetitions

Whenever you are in a learning session, repetitions have been seen to be effective. To further help in rewiring your brain, repetitions must be carried out faster than you are used to. This tends to improve your alertness and your mind is less likely to drift off the task at hand.

▷ Don't be Hard on Yourself

As long as errors do not compromise the safety, they serve as an important part of learning. Your brain does not seem to notice if you carry out a certain task correctly. If there is a mistake somewhere, you will be determined to repeat the activity until you get it right. Do not beat yourself up if you notice any errors but just keep going.

▷ Rest Intervals are Essential

Rest intervals have been seen to engage neurons in the cortex and hippocampus in a way that mimics the previous learning process ten times faster (Huberman, 2021). Clearly, rest intervals are important when it comes to rewiring your brain. Consider adding rest breaks in your learning bouts.

▷ Reward Yourself

Rewards are helpful whenever there is a need for motivation. By using intermittent rewards, your motivation and urge to pursue tasks become improved. Consider these once in a while.

▷ Do Shorter Learning Sessions

Whenever you are in a learning session, you may have noticed that your concentration decreases as time extends. It has been noted that an individual can maintain deep concentration and focus on learning for 90 minutes. After 90 minutes, it will be difficult to maintain focus. Therefore, consider limiting your learning sessions to 90 minutes or less.

▷ Consider a Non-Sleep Deep Rest (NSDR)

After a learning session, consider having a short nap or a non-sleep deep rest. This has been seen to improve your depth and rate of learning. Examples of NSDR that you could use are taking a brief nap of about 20 minutes or using yoga nidra.

How Music Changes the Brain

Would you like to get a total brain workout? Listen to your favorite music. It has been noted that playing or listening to music is a great tool in relation to keeping your brain engaged as you age. According to research, listening to music is associated with a reduction in blood pressure, anxiety, and pain (John Hopkins Medicine, 2022). Music has also been linked with enhanced sleep quality, memory, and mental alertness.

Do Online Games and Apps Really Work?

Millions of people worldwide have resorted to brain-training apps in order to boost their brain health. However, the benefits of these apps tend to be controversial according to scientific research. Some studies revealed the improvement of working memory, processing speed, and executive functions in young people (Sandoiu, 2018). In seniors, preservation of cognitive health has been observed. On the other hand, some researchers reported the absence of such benefits. More research in this area may help settle this issue.

FINDING PURPOSE AND DISCOVERY

It is important for you to have a purpose in life. When you discover your purpose, numerous things start falling into place. There are many benefits that are linked to having a purpose in life. Read on to get more information.

Having a Life Purpose is Linked to Better Brain Health

Having a purpose is associated with increased brain health, reduced dementia, and lowered cognitive impairment. Research has suggested that psychological well-being can slow cognitive deterioration (Rice, 2022). By all means, consider finding your purpose in life.

The Difference Between Purpose and Happiness

When looking at the two words, *purpose* is primarily associated with meaning, whereas *happiness* is commonly linked to satisfaction. However, happiness sensations can be grouped into two types, eudemonic and hedonic. The following sections will provide more information.

▷ Eudemonic Pursuits

Through meaning or purpose, eudemonic pursuits are able to meet certain human needs. For example, older adults tend to find meaning in strengthening interpersonal relationships. By finding a purpose in cementing your relationships with others, other health behaviors that help protect your body and brain are subsequently promoted.

▷ Hedonic Pursuits

Unlike eudaimonic pursuits, hedonic pursuits are more about satisfying oneself. Hedonic pursuits bring happiness by satisfying your urges or needs. Sometimes, this type of happiness can incorporate mindless or unhealthy behaviors such as overindulgence.

The Relationship of Science and Living With Purpose

Due to research, it is now known that there is a relationship between science and living with a purpose.

This was revealed by a study carried out in 2022 that as you age, life satisfaction also improves due to the increased release of oxytocin (Rice, 2022). There is likely a relationship between purpose and meaning with major dementia-related biomarkers. These biomarkers include cellular stress response and neuroinflammation.

LIFESTYLES FOR BRAIN FUNCTION IMPROVEMENT

Exercise has been proven to be good for both the brain and the body. Social connectedness and physical activity have been mentioned by research as being helpful in relation to preventing cognitive decline (Rice, 2022). Adopting a healthy lifestyle is more likely to increase your life expectancy and lower your chance of developing Alzheimer's disease. Results from a certain study suggested that your ability to manage cholesterol and glucose during your early childhood can help reduce the chance of Alzheimer's disease.

You may have noticed that if you are driven by a certain purpose in life, your mind is more likely to be stimulated. In addition to that, your physical well-being tends to be enhanced as well. This section will highlight some of the ways that you could utilize to enhance your brain health.

Consider Engaging in Volunteer Work

Volunteer work is one way you could use to promote your brain health. If volunteering provides purpose to your life, you could consider putting more hours into it. By volunteering, you tend to connect and socialize with other people who are passionate about similar causes.

Spend More Time Outside

Consider spending more time outside if you want to boost your brain health. A study that was carried out in 2021 found that being outside in nature has benefits such as enhanced thinking, memory, and concentration. You will also notice that outdoor activities help to inspire social connections with others.

Prioritize Your Relationships

One of the longest studies carried out at Harvard University established a link between meaningful relationships and longevity. Instances of depression and Alzheimer's disease tend to be less in people who nurture their relationships with friends, community, and family. Therefore, it is crucial to prioritize your relationships.

BENEFITS OF HAVING A SENSE OF PURPOSE

It has been noted that determining your goal or aim in life helps you in having a sense of purpose. This has been scientifically proven to provide physical and psychological benefits. Possessing a sense of purpose helps in giving your life a meaning. Also, it allows you to make a positive contribution in other people's lives. Let's take a look at the benefits of having a sense of purpose in this section.

Helps Prevent Dementia

Your purpose in life has an impact on your central nervous system. There is a study that was carried out over a period of seven years, on nine hundred older people who were at risk of developing dementia. The study revealed a 50 percent less chance of developing Alzheimer's for people who possessed a purpose as opposed to those who had a low purpose.

Increases Happiness

There is a certain happiness that comes with having a purpose in life. It has been scientifically proven that people who lack purpose in life tend to suffer from anxiety, loneliness, boredom, and depression. If you are aware of your purpose, it is not new knowledge to you to understand that living by what you value makes you happier.

Reduces the Risk of Heart Attack and Stroke

It is interesting to note that goal-orientation is directly linked to stroke and heart attack. According to research, if you have a purpose in life, you will subsequently have a reduced risk of stroke and heart attack. By having a reduced risk of these diseases, you also tend to have a decreased risk of frailty and mortality. Research revealed a 22 percent reduced stroke risk for older adults. In another study, a 27 percent decrease in heart attack was seen in people who have a purpose in life (virtuesforlife.com, 2022).

Reduces Sleep Disturbances

Sleep is mainly associated with laziness, but it is important to note that it is a necessity to have adequate sleep. Individuals who have low purpose usually experience disturbances in their sleep. You may be interested to note that people who have a strong sense of purpose have a 16 percent reduction in experiencing sleep disturbances. This may be because, as they achieve their meaningful goals, their stress levels are likely lower.

Is Linked to Greater job Satisfaction

A study that included hospital service workers revealed that those who merely considered themselves as cleaning staff possessed less job satisfaction (virtuesfor-life.com, 2022). This was contrary to those who considered themselves as part of the team that assisted in healing patients. Having this positive thought provided them with more meaning in relation to their work.

Has a Positive Effect on Academics

It may be commonly expected that having a purpose in life has a positive effect on academics. A study revealed that adolescents who possessed a sense of purpose in life had enhanced academic performance as opposed to those who did not. Students with higher purpose also find academic studies more meaningful.

HOW TO PRACTICE PURPOSE

There are numerous ways to find your purpose in life. It is also helpful to determine what provides you a sense of ambition. Some may discover their purpose through going on a quest. Let's discuss some of the ways that you can utilize to practice your purpose.

Determine What Provides You with a Sense of Purpose in Life

To help you determine what it is that provides you with a sense of meaning, there are questions that you have to ask yourself. For instance, "What are your talents and skills?"; "What is of importance to you?"; "What brings meaning to your life?" You will have clarity once you determine the answers to these questions. In case you already know your purpose, it is helpful for you to look for ways in which you could expand it.

Go on a Quest

By going on a mission or an adventure, your aim can be brought to life. Take time to think about the quest you would like to tackle. Afterward, take action and see how it goes.

Prioritize Your Purpose

You are on the right track if you have defined your objective. Working toward this objective should be at the center of all your activities. Whenever you can and wherever you go it is better for you to always consider putting your purpose first.

IMPROVING YOUR MEMORY

You may be wondering how you could improve your memory. The good news is that there are a variety of options. More details are provided in the "how to" part in this section.

To improve your memory, avoid multitasking because it lowers your brain efficiency. When multitasking, you tend to force your brain to move from one mission to another. Another way to improve your memory is to set time limits. It is helpful to give yourself some time on which you get to work on a specific task. Take regular breaks and include deadlines. Removing distractions is another way you could use to enhance your memory. For example, organizing your workspace.

In case you want to remember something, consider doing self-testing. You can do this by developing and answering questions related to your topic of interest. Hacking your brain is another way to improve your memory. Your brain is more likely to remember certain elements as opposed to others. To hack your brain, it helps to perform rehearsals and make connections. Making connections can mean drawing a relationship tree on a paper or putting them in a hierarchy.

KNOW YOUR WHY

We have established that you have to know your why. Reasons have been given as to why you should know your purpose. Here is a questionnaire that we recommend you answer truthfully.

1. What inspires you?
2. What are your natural strengths?
3. What makes you happy?
4. What are your regrets?
5. Do you consider yourself a good person?
6. What are the four things that you love about yourself?
7. What do you like to do in your free time?

Maintaining the neuroplasticity of your brain is a crucial part of taking care of this organ. The same applies with developing a sense of purpose. In both cases the health and functionality of your brain is enhanced. Cultivating a sense of purpose also improves the quality and quantity of your sleep. Learn more about the role of sleep in promoting brain health in the next chapter.

6

THE IMPORTANCE OF SLEEP AND RELAXATION

Sleep is the golden chain that ties health and our bodies together.

— THOMAS DEKKER

For many years, the brain has been a mystery to both scientists and psychologists, but one thing that all parties can agree on is the critical role it plays in the body. You need to take care of your brain, and one of the ways to do that is to sleep. Sleep allows your brain to rejuvenate and stay healthy so that when you wake up you are ready to tackle whatever challenges come your way. In this chapter, we will dive deeper into how sleep works and its functions in keeping your brain happy and healthy.

Sleep issues affect anyone and everyone around the world, regardless of age, gender, or ethnicity. In America, studies have shown that half of the population noted that they felt drowsiness three to seven days a week (Suni, 2021). The most significant contribution to this is failure to get adequate sleep. According to studies, you need an uninterrupted seven to nine hours of sleep each night (Suni, 2021). However, according to a survey that was done by the Sleep Foundation, it was found that in the US, 35.2% of adults reported getting an average of fewer than seven hours of sleep per night (Suni, 2021).

WHAT IS SLEEP?

Sleep is a naturally occurring activity in every living creature. In the past, sleep was conceived as a passive ritual in which we simply close our eyes and thoughts and then open them feeling rejuvenated after a few hours. Modern studies have shown that our brains remain active, doing some housekeeping when the rest of the body is getting some rest. The physical, mental and emotional benefits of sleep are known by the majority of people all around the world, but the biological functions of sleep are still a mystery to many. Scientists have, however, identified all the parts of the brain that are essential when it comes to sleeping and relaxing.

THE ANATOMY OF SLEEP

Found within the brain, is the small hypothalamus. This organ has multiple nerve cell groupings that control sleep and arousal. The hypothalamus contains the Suprachiasmatic nucleus (SCN), which are thousands of cells found in compounds, responsible for controlling your behavioral rhythms from receiving and processing light information. The brain stem is another structure found at the base of the brain. It communicates with the hypothalamus to control the transitions of cycles that occur between sleeping and waking up. The thalamus acts as a relay for sensory information, sending it to the cerebral cortex, which interprets and organizes the message into either short or long-term memory.

The pineal gland is found within the two hemispheres of the brain and its main function is to produce melatonin, which is a hormone that helps you find sleep after the lights dim. The basal forebrain is located near the front bottom part of the brain. It promotes sleep through the release of adenosine, which stimulates your sleep drive. The amygdala is a tiny structure in the brain that aids in processing emotions and is mostly active during the Rapid Eye Movement (REM) sleep cycle.

SLEEP STAGES

When you sleep, you pass through two types of sleep cycles, which are Rapid Eye Movement (REM) sleep and non-REM sleep. Non-REM sleep contributes to the four out of the five stages of sleep that exist while REM sleep is the last cycle.

- **Stage one:** This is known as light sleep and is the stage where you drift in and out of sleep and can easily be awoken. Your entire body relaxes, and involuntary body activities such as the heartbeat, eye movement, and brain waves slow down.
- **Stage two:** This describes the window between light and deep sleep. Your body will be preparing itself to enter deep sleep, and it does so by halting eye movement and enhancing muscles transition between contracting and

relaxing. The brain waves become slower and your body temperature lowers.

- **Stages three and four:** At this point, you would have entered deep sleep. The brain waves slow down and are interspersed with shorter, faster waves. These are called delta waves. There is no eye movement or muscle activity and you cannot be easily awakened during these stages.
- **Stage five:** This is the last stage, also called REM sleep. This stage reintroduces rapid breathing, and increased eye movements, heart rate, and blood pressure are experienced. Your muscles are temporarily paralyzed.

SLEEP MECHANISMS

Your body has two biological mechanisms that remain active as you sleep. These are the Circadian Rhythms and Homeostasis. According to the American Sleep Association, Circadian Rhythms can be defined as the regular changes in your body's mental and physical characteristics that happen throughout the course of the day (American Sleep Association, 2018). Your body's own biological "clock" is responsible for controlling the majority of circadian rhythms through environmental cues such as light and temperature.

The sleep-wake homeostasis is the second sleep mechanism that is active when you close your eyes and this mechanism keeps track of your sleep drive. The homeopathic sleep drive regulates sleep intensity and actively reminds your body when it needs to sleep. Many factors influence your sleep-wake requirements, including medical conditions, medications, stress, sleep environments, and your diet. One of the biggest influences on your sleep-wake needs is light exposure and this is where homeostasis and the Circadian rhythm intersect.

SLEEP DURATION

A multitude of factors, including age, influence the amount of sleep required by each individual. Infants tend to sleep longer, requiring approximately sixteen hours of sleep each day. The long hours may help with proper development and brain growth. Teenagers usually require approximately nine hours whereas most adult sleep needs range between seven to eight hours per night. With adults, other influencing factors such as longer work hours, round-the-clock entertainment, and other activities play a role in people getting less sleep. Such factors explain the fluctuations in sleeping hours with some needing as little as four hours, whereas others may need as much as ten hours per night.

Pregnant women also tend to frequently need additional hours of sleep, especially during the first three months. The older you get, the lighter, and shorter you tend to sleep while still requiring the same sleep time frame as you did in your early adulthood. As a result, an increasing number of senior citizens are turning to sleep-inducing medications in order to get a good night's sleep.

DREAMING

Everyone dreams. You dream for roughly two hours every night, though they may be very difficult to remember. The exact purpose of dreaming is unknown. However, some psychologists believe that dreams are a way of channeling and processing your emotions. Your dreams will most likely be a reflection of your day's thoughts and events.

The amount of sleep you require may also be influenced by genes. These genes include the ones that regulate neuron excitability as well as "clock" genes, which govern your circadian cycles and sleep schedule. Sleep problems have often been linked to specific regions on several chromosomes, according to genome-wide association studies (Dashti et al, 2019). Between sleep and wake, the levels of expression of certain genes expressed in the cerebral cortex and other areas of the brain alter. If you feel like you have a sleep disorder and want to get a diagnosis, a polysomnogram may be the way to go. A polysomnogram is a sleep study that records your brain's waves, blood oxygen levels, heart rate, and breathing. This will require you to spend the night in the laboratory where they can track these parameters and the acquired data is used to determine how you go through the sleep stages.

THE BRAIN AND SLEEP DEPRIVATION

Sleep is an opportunity for your brain to recover from all the negative situations and thoughts you process when you are awake. During sleep, your brain stores new information and releases some of it as unnecessary. Communication between nerve cells continues while you sleep. As you sleep, the brain's glymphatic system is initiated, which clears waste from the central nervous system, allowing your brain to work better when you wake up. Memory, problem-solving, creativity, and judgment are among the brain functions that are amplified by a good night's sleep.

Sleep is also essential in allowing the brain to increase activity in the areas that regulate emotions, thereby sustaining emotional health. While brain activity diminishes during the non-REM periods, some brain waves continue to pulse. The third stage of non-REM sleep is marked by a reduction in brain activity, but some brain waves will continue to be visible. REM sleep contrasts with non-REM sleep by showing large signs of brain activity, comparable to what happens when you are awake. To coordinate rest and recovery, the brain activates and deactivates different chemicals at different times.

Sleep deprivation brings forth highly damaging effects on your brain and cognitive function. When you do not have a healthy sleep pattern, your brain will have difficulties performing the functions it normally undertakes as you sleep. Unhealthy sleep patterns are usually characterized by short, interrupted, or fragmented nights.

Short-Term Effects

Sleep deprivation has a wide range of potential short-term effects on cognitive performance. It can reduce your attention and learning acumen through symptoms such as lethargy and exhaustion. You may unintentionally dose off for a few seconds as a result, a phenomenon that is widely known as microsleep. Daytime lethargy can cause substantial cognitive problems by showing symptoms that are comparable to being drunk. Such symptoms include slow thinking and reduced reaction time.

Lack of, or interrupted sleep, causes more injury to specific sections of the brain and this has varying impacts on different types of cognition such as decision making. Sleepiness lowers judgment and making decisions is more challenging as you are unable to accurately assess situations and react appropriately. There has also been significant evidence that sleep and memory are intertwined (McCarley, 2007). REM and non-REM sleep cycles are needed for memory consolidation, with the latter being responsible for the storage of facts and events. REM sleep is responsible for remembering actions and skills. When both of these cycles do not reach completion, you may begin to develop false memories.

Individuals deprived of proper sleep experience problems with the ability to follow instructions. Without enough sleep, motor abilities, rhythm, and even some forms of speech may deteriorate. Not sleeping well reduces your brain's ability to recognize and successfully adapt to unfamiliar situations. Sleep deprivation has also been shown to reduce cognitive flexibility, thereby limiting one's ability to adapt and thrive in uncertain, changing situations. Sleep deprivation results in rigid thinking and "feedback blunting," which reduces your ability to learn.

Lack of sleep alters how emotional information is processed. Normally, recognizing the emotional context of things is often vital when learning something new, assessing a situation, or making a decision. Inadequate sleep, which negatively impacts mood, makes it difficult for you to adequately digest any emotional components of information. The altered emotional response hinders judgment in many circumstances. Another element of cognition that is damaged by sleep deficit is creativity. As you sleep, your brain organizes your new ideas and thoughts hence, your ability to be creative and imaginative is amplified by having a healthy sleep pattern.

Sleep deprivation or restlessness might have an indirect impact on cognition as a result of the other issues that it creates. If you struggle with heavy headaches or migraines, not sleeping well could aggravate the situation. You might have to deal with dizziness and headaches every morning. Mental illnesses such as anxiety and depression tend to worsen when you do not allow yourself some time to rest. Existing studies substantially support the idea that insufficient sleep hinders effective thinking. If you do not get enough sleep, you are more prone to make mistakes, forget new information, have memory problems, and make poor decisions. This can negatively impact your intellectual performance, scholastic accomplishments, creative endeavors, and workplace efficiency. You may put your health at risk as well. Many accidents have been caused by sleepy drivers and some people lost their limbs while operating dangerous machines whilst half asleep.

Long-Term Effects

The most common effects of poor sleep are the ones that show immediate symptoms, but recent studies show that insufficient sleep damages your brain in the long run (Verdile et al, 2004). Sleep aids the brain in doing crucial housekeeping tasks, such as removing harmful chemicals and when this task is not regularly achieved, these chemical residues will build up and deteriorate cognitive function, causing mental disorders such as Alzheimer's dementia. Alzheimer's dementia is caused by beta-amyloid, which builds up when the brain is not able to perform waste disposal. If you already suffer from a mental disorder, high chances are that inadequate sleep will worsen the symptoms (Verdile et al, 2004).

Sleep deprivation affects everyone differently. Adults tend to suffer less in the long run, as compared to teenagers who still have a growing brain. Sleep disorders such as insomnia and obstructive sleep apnea are some of the reasons why you could be having poor sleep patterns. Insomnia has been linked to many issues concerning normal brain functions, including loss of concentration and irritability. Obstructive Sleep Apnea is a sleep disorder where you have trouble breathing throughout the night due to blocked airways. You may also struggle to find sleep as a result of these symptoms.

IS TOO MUCH SLEEP GOOD?

Getting too much sleep may not be good for your brain function as well. Oversleeping may be caused by suffering from a disease where one of the symptoms is a lack of energy and fatigue. Studies have shown that oversleeping may result in the reduction of brain efficiency, likening the effects to that of a person who has just woken up from a coma (Erickson, 2020).

Improved sleep is the most practical strategy if you are suffering from sleep disorders to improve your cognitive performance. Good sleep is your best bet in the long run, from keeping your brain healthy and working to helping you prevent life-threatening diseases and situations.

BENEFITS OF GOOD SLEEP

Falling asleep is not rocket science. Sleeping may be difficult for many but it does not have to be for you. There are a number of benefits to actually getting an adequate amount of sleep.

Enhances Better Mood

According to scientists, those who go to bed late are more likely to be overwhelmed by negative thoughts (Guadagni et al, 2014). So, focusing on good sleep habits can help your mood, considering that you may worry less. You may find yourself becoming friendlier. People who get little to no sleep, tend to be more irritable and short-tempered. Try going to sleep a little earlier and experience the benefits to your social interactions. You may even become a safer driver. A high percentage of people have admitted to driving on the road with some sort of sleep deprivation and actually falling asleep at the wheel. To make sure you reduce the risk of an accident and that you always get to your destination on time and one piece, please, get a healthy amount of sleep.

Improved Appearance

Sleeping early might help you to actually look better. People who do not get enough do not look as good.

Sleep-deprived adults were judged as less attractive, less healthy, less accessible, and sadder than well-rested people when participants saw photographs of them (Sundelin et al, 2017).

Stronger Immune System

Getting a good night's sleep could also help you avoid getting the flu among other diseases. Getting enough rest strengthens your immune system, thereby protecting you against viruses in the air and speeding up your recovery time if you do become infected.

HOW TO IMPROVE YOUR SLEEP

Falling asleep is not always easy, especially if you already have problems with insomnia. However, this does not mean there are no ways to help you. There are a couple of suggestions to fast-track your journey to falling asleep peacefully and healthily and we will explore some of them in this section.

- **Create a sleep pattern that is unique to you:** Make a night time routine and make sure you adhere to it diligently. It will become easier and more natural to maintain your sleep rhythm once your body has found it.

- **Start going to bed early:** According to experts, the best time to fall asleep is between 10:00 p.m. and 2:00 a.m. (Tekeli, 2017). This is the pattern that your circadian clock follows, So, if you want to sleep better, rearrange your schedule such that you are in bed by 9:30 p.m.

- **Put on your pajamas:** Changing into sleep-only clothing is an important aspect of a fantastic sleep ritual. It is an element of the emotional and mental preparation that helps you fall asleep.

- **Try stretching your jaw before you sleep:** Many people have a lot of tightness in their jaw, which may sound strange. Pull your lips open with your index and middle fingers on each hand and massage the upper jaw area around your ears with these fingers. Make little circles with your fingertips behind the earlobes by pressing softly. It may be slightly painful but it will be like having your own personal massage therapist and it greatly helps your body to relax.

- **Try breathing through your left nostril:** Deep breathing is used in almost all relaxation treatments. Close your right nostril and breathe for two to three minutes before lying down. Your body's parasympathetic nerve system, or rest and digest system, will naturally engage, allowing you to sleep more easily.

- **Take warm baths every night before you sleep:** Do this every night until you have established a functioning sleep routine. Dim the lights and put on soothing music while you are in the tub, this will relax you and also send the messages to your body that you are ready to wind down.

- **Run cold on your feet:** Does this sound unconventional? Yes, but it is very helpful if you are trying to sleep. The physical jolt of cold water helps your body breathe better and it encourages your body to naturally work harder to stay warm, thereby increasing your oxygen intake.

- **Apply sleep meditation to your routine:** There is a wonderful kundalini meditation that might help you relax and sleep. However, before you do it, you have to make sure your posture is correct by sitting tall. Your hands should be on your lap with the palms facing up, and thumb tips facing forward and away from the body. Your eyes should focus on the tip of your nose, and as you do the breathing technique, you mentally chant the mantra, "Sa-Ta-Na-Ma."

- **Before going to bed, drink a glass of water:**
  When you sleep, you become dehydrated, and
  this may lead you to have a restless night or
  cause you to wake up. If you do get up during
  the night, try keeping the bathroom lights off
  and return to bed as soon as you are finished.
  You could also consider using sleep-related
  apps. Not a novel idea, but one worth exploring
  if you weigh the benefits and the drawbacks.
- **Limit daytime naps to less than ninety
  minutes or do not nap at all:** This will help
  you adhere to your sleep schedule and not
  interfere with it.

YOGA NIDRA

Yoga in general has been widely recommended for its
benefits, but the thought of flowing and holding poses
is not very appealing to most people. Yoga nidra is a
style of yoga that you can do by just lying on your bed.
It can help you feel relaxed and refreshed. According to
a Yoga therapist and yoga program manager Judy Bar,
in yoga nidra, you lie down with the intention of
moving into a profound level of conscious awareness
sleep, which is a more relaxed state of awareness
(Kumar, 2008). It entails transitioning from awake
consciousness to dreaming, then to not dreaming while

still awake, basically shifting from the unconscious to the conscious state.

Yoga nidra works with the autonomic nervous system, responsible for controlling bodily functions that occur without conscious effort. The sympathetic and parasympathetic nervous systems are also part of this system. According to Bar, meditation is practiced to calm the sympathetic system and stimulate the parasympathetic more. When you have reached a healthy balance at a macro level, the pineal gland will be stimulated to release melatonin, a hormone that plays a crucial role in enhancing sleep. Yoga Nidra has cognitive benefits, in addition to reducing anxiety. Yoga Nidra can also come in handy when you can't take longer naps during the day.

Please note that procedures for Yoga Nidra are available on YouTube for free. You can, therefore, follow these steps and enjoy the benefits of Yoga Nidra on your brain. The link below will take you to a good YouTube video for Yoga Nidra on https://www.youtube.com/watch?v=M0u9GST_j3s&t=48s.

DAYTIME REST AND RELAXATION

Your brain needs to relax and get some downtime even when you are awake. Downtime replenishes the brain's attention and promotes productivity and creativity. It is also necessary for you to achieve peak levels of performance. A wandering mind frees you from the confines of time, allowing us to learn from the past and make plans for the future. It may even be important to take a break from time to time to keep your moral compass in functioning order and maintain your sense of self.

Here are five easy ways in which your brain can get some downtime:

- **Prioritize sleep:** When it comes to resetting your mental health, sleep comes first and is effective.
- **Start a new project:** Many people do not welcome change, yet switching your routine or introducing something new into your life might provide your brain with the needed refreshment.
- **Mind your mind**: It can be very difficult to slow down, but taking time to practice mindfulness, journal your thoughts, and meditate will prove helpful when resetting your mental health.
- **Get some fresh air every day**: A simple pleasure, such as exposure to the vast outdoors, might sometimes be the key to being happy.

- **Give yourself a brain dump:** Write down all your ideas, fears, questions, needs, wants, and all other things that may occupy your thoughts. This can really help you clear your mind, organize your thoughts and help you regain control.

Your brain has many components and many functions in the body and taking care of it should be a conscious decision that you make every day. The best way to keep mentally healthy is by getting a good amount of sleep, and taking some time to relax and refresh. Another good way to keep your brain healthy and happy is by making good social connections as discussed in the next chapter.

CREATE MEANINGFUL CONNECTIONS

Social connection is such a basic feature of human experience that when we are deprived of it, we suffer.

— LEONARD MLODINOW

When my father was suffering from dementia, all the members of our family took part in taking good care of him. From this experience, I realized the value of social connections in dealing with dementia. The people who were close to and around my father were positively contributing to his ability to go through his condition. Based on this, the main focus of this chapter is to explore social connections and how they relate to brain and cognitive health.

SOCIAL CONNECTIONS: AN OVERVIEW

Social connections describe the relationships that people have with each other. Social connections can either be close or distant. Your family and friends are good examples of close connections that people have with each other. Those people that you communicate with on a casual basis are part of your distant social connections circle. Please note that being a close or distant connection has nothing to do with the physical distance between you. For instance, your next-door neighbor could be a distant connection. On the other hand, a family member who is on another continent could be your closest association, even though you can only communicate through the internet or tele-phonically.

The importance of social connection is mainly in the idea of being there for each other. The people around you can help you to enjoy your great moments. When things get bad, they can give you a shoulder to lean on and give you strength. Simply put, being linked to the people around you contributes to your resilience. We can define resilience as the extent to which you are able to bounce back after going through difficult situations. Note that not all connections can make you more resilient, but positive ones do. Surrounding yourself with people who have a positive outlook on life will give you the strength to face and tackle the challenges of life. Mind you, positivity and negativity are contagious.

You can view resilience as "borrowed power or strength." It's like you can use the abilities of your friends and other people around you when yours might possibly fail you. The associations that you have with other people can contribute to how you manage your feelings. Generally, the stronger and more positive the connections are, the greater the possibility of being emotionally stable. Your mind registers more security when you have reliable people who are available to support you.

BENEFITS OF BUILDING HEALTHY SOCIAL CONNECTIONS

There are even more benefits that are associated with high social connection and we will discuss some of them in this section. Here are some good things that you may gain after building positive associations:

- **Longevity:** It is reported that people who have high social connections increase the probability of living for more years by 50% (Seppala, 2014). One of the explanations for this possible result is reduced depression. When you have people around you, the risks of some mental issues such as anxiety and stress are significantly reduced. Just the fact that you have some people to share your troubles with will go a long way.

- **Increased immunity:** People who are well connected express the gene for immunity more. A study that was one by Steve Cole revealed that the gene that is affected by loneliness is the same that is responsible for coding inflammation and immune function (Seppala, 2014). Therefore, if that gene is not dealing with loneliness, then it becomes more oriented to enhancing your immunity. This can be done by building and increasing your connections.

- **Higher esteem and empathy:** Increased links with other people are associated with higher levels of confidence and empathy. By continuously talking to other people, you tend to learn more about various personalities. Such experience elevates the way you understand the people around you, and this is referred to as empathy. Just knowing that there is someone who cares boosts your self-esteem.

- **Positive feedback loop:** Have you ever realized that the people whom you trust and cooperate with tend to return the same favor to you? This is what we are referring to as the positive feedback loop. In other words, social connections create an environment where you can share vibes of social, emotional, and physical wellbeing with the people around you.

DANGERS ASSOCIATED WITH LOW SOCIAL CONNECTIONS

Avoiding building and maintaining healthy associations has dangers that come with it. Some of these negative effects can be quite detrimental as you will see in this section. The dangers of absent, low, or poor connections include the following:

- **Negatively affects your health:** Did you know that the negative effects of low social connections are worse than high blood pressure, smoking, and obesity? Therefore, the more you reduce social connections, the more you deprive yourself of good health.

- **Increased susceptibility to anxiety and depression:** As we alluded to earlier, the more you interact with other people, the less likely you are to deal with depression and anxiety issues. Your social connections will enhance your emotional, social, and psychological resilience.
- **Higher inflammation:** Low social connections are linked with increased inflammation at the cellular level.
- **Increased orientation toward violence and other antisocial behavior:** When you don't have many social connections, your empathy is more likely to be low. This can create more of an "I don't care" kind of attitude, which is usually supportive of various forms of antisocial behaviors, including violence.
- **Slower recovery from disease:** People who are not well-connected tend to take longer to recover when they get sick. This could also be because they lack the resilience and elevated immunity that comes with creating positive connections.
- **Suicide:** In worst-case scenarios, people take their lives when they have little to no links with other people. This is primarily because they

might feel as if no one cares. Without people around you, you may lack love.

THE SECRET TO A LONGER LIFE

The contribution that positive social connections have to longevity is immense. Most of the senior citizens that you probably admire today are not there because they were strong enough to beat ailments such as heart diseases and cancer. If you were to hold a survey, you would realize that most of them have one thing in common, strong, healthy, and positive social connections. Howard S. Friedman, a psychologist at the University of California co-authored a book titled *"The Longevity Project."* In an interview about this book, Friedman highlighted the importance of social interactions in various sectors of an individual's life including marriage, family, friendship, and religious observance (Novotney, 2022).

In response to the question, "What is the most surprising finding in your research?" Friedman alluded that it was the fact that the susceptibility to diseases and injury is different for all individuals. More interestingly, Friedman explained that much of the differences are due to social relations that are reflected in marriages, friendships, and families. He also highlighted these interactions work hand-in-hand with other factors in determining the level of susceptibility to diseases.

Another interesting finding that Friedman mentioned was that the strongest social predictor for shorter lifespans is the divorce between parents during childhood. This is partly because parental divorce makes children vulnerable to lifestyles that are unhealthy. For example, such children can end up smoking and drinking. They might even divorce when they get married as well.

Friedman also talked about the role of marriages in enhancing healthy, longer life. He blatantly spoke against the common adage that says, "Get married and you will live longer" (Novotney, 2022). He highlighted that this adage is only true to a few men who enjoyed good marriages and those who were truly suited for such a union. For the rest of them, marriages involved many complications, most of which would actually negatively affect longevity. Divorced men who decided to stay alone seemed to have significantly reduced lifespans. Contrastingly, women who got divorced from their troublesome husbands were healthier and more oriented toward longer lives. The same applies to those who were widowed, they did very well.

HOW SOCIAL LIFE CONTRIBUTES TO LONGEVITY

Now that you have learned that social interactions may contribute to longevity, you might be wondering how this happens. We have touched on some of these "how" aspects in passing. In this section, you will learn more about how your social life positively impacts your lifespan.

Your Social Life and the Brain

All the biological processes that take place in your body are linked to the brain. Let's take the example of when you are stressed, the brain triggers the increased release of the hormone called cortisol. This hormone causes your cardiovascular system to activate the "fight or flight" response. When you create strong relationships, you can reduce the chances of being stressed so the brain won't have to activate the fight or flight response.

Loneliness has been reported to be one of the stressors that trigger the brain into action. This stressor not only increases the production of cortisol in your body but also promotes inflammation. Unfortunately, both inflammation and cortisol have detrimental effects on your health in the long run.

Social interaction triggers the secretion of different hormones from those that are triggered by loneliness and stress. For instance, when you communicate with others in meaningful relationships, oxytocin is released. In addition, to reduce pain and cortisol levels, oxytocin improves your brain's response to stressors. Oxytocin also contributes to the growth of new brain cells. Interestingly, some of the gestures that are usually involved when people interact have been reported to increase oxytocin secretion in the human body. These include hugs and eye contact. Some research has shown that even eye contact with your dog can increase the production of oxytocin (Nagasawa et al., 2015). One study investigated the effects of social interactions on about 7,000 participants over a period of nine years (Berkman and Syme, 1979). The results of the study showed that individuals who had more social ties live longer than those who didn't.

Creating Healthy Habits

Human beings learn continuously, even from their connections. When you associate yourself with positive people, you can learn new habits that help you to live longer. These include eating well and exercising. Instead of just looking at how you can benefit from social relationships, try to make the connections mutually beneficial. Social interactions give you the opportunity to put a smile on someone's face by being there for them. It doesn't have to be face-t0-face all the time, phone calls and text messages will also do. Play some games with others and engage in other social activities, including dancing together with others.

See Beyond the Individual Benefits

While the benefits of social connections are often measured at the individual level, it is vital to find out how they help the community of which you are part. According to research, a community that is made up of people who socially interact has a lesser risk of diseases like cardiovascular disease and diabetes, overall (Hopper, 2020). This means that the individuals who make up such a community will be healthier. This contributes to longevity. Therefore, anything that contributes to a socially interactive community contributes toward this cause. This includes visiting senior citizens and simply creating a fearless and safe community with crime levels that are as low as possible.

RECOMMENDATIONS FOR PROMOTING MEANINGFUL ENGAGEMENTS

When it comes to developing meaningful engagements, there is no "one size fits all" strategy. People connect and get the best out of their associations in various ways. Sometimes, the way people engage is influenced by other factors, some of which are gender, past associations, personalities, culture, individual preferences, and context. Regardless of all these factors, this section will allude to different methods that you can employ for creating meaningful engagements.

Focus on What You Enjoy

You can easily connect with other people when you are happier. Therefore, getting involved in activities that you love can create a good atmosphere for creating positive relationships. If you love basketball, taking part in the sport can see you meeting new people or maintaining good relationships with the ones that you already know. Identify what you love and go for it. There is a high probability that there are other people who love it, too and that common ground can be a basis for continuous interaction.

Turn to Professionals

You might not find people around you to start associations. Technology can be of help in such scenarios. You can use telephones and chat options on the internet to get in touch with professionals from different fields. For example, you can talk to religious leaders, free counselors, or even experts in drop-in centers. The options are endless.

Maximize Every Opportunity for Creating Connections

There is no limit on the type of connections that you should foster. This then means that you can start interacting anywhere and at any time. When you go to the movie house, why not say, "Hello" to the person sitting next to you and begin a conversation? If you go for a picnic, why not invite another family and build deeper relationships? You can attend conferences that align with your area of expertise so that you get connected to relevant people in that regard. Join support groups whose focus matches something that you are interested in. Any situation where you can possibly talk to other people is an opportunity for connection, so grab it.

Find Your Way Around Barriers to Connecting

We cannot deny the fact that barriers such as unsafe neighborhoods can hinder your zeal to build meaningful associations. However, you have to find your way around them.

One of the ways through which you can do this is by identifying someone whom you can ask for assistance. Such a person can link you to some people so that you don't lose out on building connections.

Develop Support Outside Intimate Relationship

If you are in a good intimate relationship or marriage, there is no harm in also reaching out for other connections. These will give you further support, security, and resilience. Create friendships, associations around expertise, and volunteering endeavors that foster connections. Volunteering can be done through formal organizations or informally. Local libraries are always looking for volunteers. You could visit a colleague or senior citizen in your neighborhood and help them with maintaining their garden.

Engage With Family, Friends, and Neighbors

The people who are always around you are your first chance for creating meaningful connections. Before you think of associating with other members of your community and beyond, have a circle of friends, family members, and neighbors with whom you are well linked. If your family and friends are far away, emails, phones, and video calls will help. These are some of the people who you can create close ties with. They can also help you to connect with their circle of interactions so that you widen your links. Among your close connections, try to have at least one confidante. This should be someone who you can trust. Communicate with this person or people regularly.

Connect Across Ages

Avoid limiting your connections to people who are around the same age as you. Associate with people from different age groups, even the younger children. If you have grandchildren, keep in touch with them. You can pass on some skills that you have mastered over the years to them so that they can continue with your legacy. Such skills include event management, cooking, stock market investing, baking, and creative gardening. You can even volunteer at a local school in your community just to keep in touch with the younger souls.

Try New Activities

How about trying something that you have not done before? This could be a new activity or attending an event that you normally wouldn't be part of. Consider taking a walk to the park where you can possibly meet new people and connect. You can even challenge yourself to register in political organizations, religious gatherings, as well as academic or practical courses. If you are a socially active individual, try to think of something new that you can introduce into your community. One of the most popular activities is "Pickleball." This game somewhat resembles tennis in that it is played on a court with a net. However, pickleball uses wooden paddles and a plastic ball. Organizations for those over

50, and for all ages, are popping up across the country. Another example would be to create a "workout group" if there wasn't one in your neighborhood. You are more likely to meet new people and build sustainable relationships in the process.

THE ART OF CREATING SOCIAL BONDS

No matter how many people you meet in a day, you won't create meaningful social links if you don't master some skills. This section will focus on how to make the best out of each connecting opportunity that you get. Here are the important nuggets:

Be Grateful

We all want to associate with grateful people because they make us feel important. Therefore, if you learn to be grateful, you are more prone to having sustainable relationships with the people around you. The results from some studies showed that the positive effects that are associated with gratitude are mainly experienced when one receives thanks than when they offer the same. However, no one can receive gratitude unless someone offers it. Choose to be the one who positively impacts someone through your genuine and heartfelt "Thank you."

Introversion and Extroversion as Part of Social Homeostasis

Your brain has circuits that are responsible for driving a desire to create and sustain social bonds. This is also referred to as "social hunger" and is often associated with the production of dopamine. It is important to note that both introverts and extroverts love social interaction. The only difference between these two groups of people is that the former is more quickly satisfied socially than the latter. These differences are explained by the amount of dopamine that introverts release versus that of extroverts. Therefore, when you communicate, don't assume that extroverts are talkative while introverts are not. This can be true in some instances but note that it is not always the case.

Observe or Recall Giving and Receiving Genuine Thanks

Learn by observing others who are either giving or receiving genuine gratitude. Some neuroimaging studies revealed that by simply observing when others are receiving assistance, some prosocial circuits that boost your mood are activated (Damasio, 2014). This is because human beings are wired to assess the emotional status of others as part of their own social needs. Therefore, recalling instances where someone received help is good for your social life. If you do this about three times a week, it will become embedded in your memory so you can reap the benefits.

Merge Physiologies

Some studies have shown that when people experience the same physiological conditions, they feel closer and more attached to each other (Huberman Lab, 2021). More interestingly, other research also reported that if people listen to the same story while they are in different rooms, their hearts will begin to beat in a similar pattern (Huberman Lab, 2021). Based on this wealth of evidence, you can use sharing stories as a strategy for creating strong bonds in your connections. Watch movies or listen to music together with your colleagues, friends, family members, or other people and enjoy the social benefits of merging physiologies.

INTERACTIVE ELEMENT

When all is said and done, you need to be happy to keep your brain healthy and enjoy a long life. Take some time to watch the TED Talk on this link: https://youtu. be/8KkKuTCFvzI

Creating meaningful connections is an important element of our existence as human beings. They contribute to your physical, emotional, and psychological well-being. Lower social connections are often associated with antisocial behavior, among other things. Creating healthy relationships requires you to make efforts to either create or make use of available opportunities for interacting with other people. Being grateful and sharing moments strengthens bonds between people. Positive connections keep your brain healthier and this is true. The next chapter, "Destructive myths about the brain," will explore some untrue notions that are said about the brain and its functions.

DESTRUCTIVE MYTHS ABOUT THE BRAIN

After reading this chapter, you will understand the facts behind the destructive myths that most people have about the brain. When asked about these myths, it is surprising that some people actually believe them to be true. However, this chapter will help you in demystifying many of these myths as evidenced by research. You will be shocked to note that about two-thirds of Americans think that humans utilize only 10 percent of their brains. A poll, which included more than 2,000 Americans, determined that 65% of the participants agreed with the above-mentioned myth. This is not the only myth concerning brain health that people have. Read on to get more information about the myths surrounding brain health. This chapter outlines the myths as well as the related truths about brain functions.

MYTH NUMBER 1: YOU ONLY USE 10% OF YOUR BRAIN

This is a common myth that we talked about in the previous paragraph. Many people think that you only use a small percentage of your overall brain capacity. A new poll on brain health revealed that approximately two-thirds of Americans wrongly believe that the human race uses only 10 percent of their brains (Rettner, 2013).

The above-mentioned statement is indeed not true. According to neurologists, the brain is reportedly always functional. The brain is responsible for sending signals to your body so that you are able to walk, eat, think or do just about anything. Even reflex actions require the brain to be functional. Your brain is always rapidly firing numerous neurons. This is also true even when someone is sleeping. With this information, it is clear that the myth that humans only use 10 percent of their brains can be dismissed.

MYTH NUMBER 2: ALCOHOL KILLS BRAIN CELLS

Depending on the amount of alcohol you drink, this can be a true statement. If you drink alcohol in moderation, your brain cells cannot be killed. Nevertheless, frequent or binge drinking can damage dendrites, which are the ends of neurons. When dendrites are damaged, the ability of neurons to send messages to each other is adversely affected. Furthermore, if you are addicted to alcohol, you are more likely to develop a disorder referred to as Wernicke-Korsakoff syndrome. This disorder is characterized by loss of muscle control, weakened memory, and vision impairment.

MYTH NUMBER 3: BRAIN SIZE AFFECTS INTELLIGENCE

Without excessively thinking about it, it could seem true to say that the bigger your brain is, the more intelligent you are. However, it is important to note that it is not the size, but the number of connections that are between the brain cells that have an effect on intelligence. These connections are called synapses. The more synapses there are in the brain, the more intelligent someone is.

MYTH NUMBER 4: BEING ANALYTICAL OR CREATIVE DEPENDS ON WHETHER YOU ARE RIGHT OR LEFT-BRAINED

The notion that left-brained people are more analytical and methodical, while right-brained people are creative or artistic is a myth. Research has come in handy in terms of setting the record straight on many controversial issues. The ordinary person has come up with theories of people being right-brained or left-brained. In addition to that, they have tried to assign certain abilities to people that they perceive to be right or left-brained. Nonetheless, according to the University of Utah's scientists, the myth that you are able to predominantly utilize one side of your brain as compared to the other has been debunked (Northwestern Medicine, 2022).

MYTH NUMBER 5: BABIES EXPOSED TO CLASSICAL MUSIC END UP SMARTER

It is difficult to support or dismiss this myth. This is because although it may be true, no evidence is available to support the notion that when you play classical music to a baby, they can become smarter. To totally dismiss this myth, there is a need to carry out the necessary research.

MYTH NUMBER 6: YOUR BRAIN WORKS BETTER UNDER PRESSURE

People handle pressure differently. Another point to note is that when you have a deadline that you have to beat, you tend to be motivated to work harder. However, although the pressure pushes you to work harder, it does not mean that your brain will perform better. In actual fact, when you are under pressure, you tend to be stressed, and therefore, your brain function may be impaired. On that note, we can safely dismiss the myth that your brain works better under pressure.

MYTH NUMBER 7: BRAIN GAMES IMPROVE YOUR MEMORY AND REASONING SKILLS

The above-mentioned myth can simply be demystified by the evidence that was obtained from a study that was commissioned by the British Broadcasting Corporation. In this study, more than 8600 people that are aged between 18 and 60 years of age were asked to engage in online brain games (Northwestern Medicine, 2022). These games were designed to enhance reasoning as well as memory. Participants involved in this study were required to play the games for a total of 10 minutes per day, three times a week. After a period of six weeks, the study revealed that the participants did not show enhanced cognitive function in the tasks for which they did not train in the games.

MYTH NUMBER 8: YOUR IQ STAYS THE SAME THROUGHOUT YOUR LIFE

According to research, your IQ does not stay the same throughout your life. Your IQ tends to fluctuate as you age. With that in mind, it is also crucial to note that it is an imperfect science to measure someone's intelligence. The ability of a person to think and recall information quickly is called fluid intelligence. It has been noted that fluid intelligence reaches its peak when you are at the age of 18. It then starts to decline as you get older. On the other hand, a person's emotional intelligence is more likely to improve until they reach the age of 30.

MYTH NUMBER 9: PEOPLE HAVE DIFFERENT LEARNING STYLES

Owing to the myth that people have different learning styles, teachers tend to structure their classrooms according to their students' learning styles. However, a number of studies have indicated that no difference is present in the way people learn. The Anatomical Sciences Education Journal published data from hundreds of students who responded to surveys that required information about the type of learners they perceived themselves to be. Upon getting this information, the teachers started to structure their lessons according to the learning styles reported by the students. From this exercise, scientists unraveled that no significant improvement was present in the test scores of the students.

MYTH NUMBER 10: THE BRAIN DECLINES AS YOU GET OLDER

Just as the body eventually deteriorates with age, it would be expected that the brain also declines as you get older. However, it has been noted that although some cognitive functions deteriorate as you age, most of your mental skills become better as you grow older. When compared to younger brains, older brains perform better in relation to emotional regulation, conflict resolution, vocabulary, and comprehension.

MYTH NUMBER 11: HUMANS HAVE THE BIGGEST BRAINS

In proportion to human body size, it has been noted that the human brain is quite big. However, it is important to quickly demystify the myth that humans have the biggest brains. Actually, the adult brain measures approximately 15 centimeters in length and has a weight of about three pounds. In comparison, the sperm whale has the largest animal brain, its weight is registered at an astounding 18 pounds. We could also look at the elephant, which is around 11 pounds in average brain size.

When looking at the relative brain size in relation to body size, humans tend to be at the top of the list. However, it is inaccurate to say that humans have the largest brains. Therefore, the myth that humans have the biggest brains can safely be dismissed.

MYTH NUMBER 12: ADULTS STOP FORMING NEW BRAIN CELLS

Some people think that, as adults, they have numerous brain cells and that it is impossible for their bodies to produce new ones. They strongly think that once they lose the cells they have, they are incapable of forming new ones. According to research, it has been revealed that the hippocampus of the brain can form new cells in a process called neurogenesis. We should also mention that there is some controversy around this topic. According to the National Institute of Health, some neuroscientists are not fully satisfied that new brain cells can be formed in adults.

MYTH NUMBER 13: THERE ARE 100 BILLION NEURONS IN THE HUMAN BRAIN

This commonly stated statistic has been repeated for such a long period of time that its origins have become unclear. To uncover the reality behind the number of neurons in the human brain, research was carried out in 2009 (Cherry, 2021). The researcher counted the neurons in adult brains and discovered that the number that had been commonly popular was a bit away from the true value. According to this research, it has been noted that the human brain has approximately 85 billion neurons. Results from this research allow us to safely dismiss the myth that there are 100 billion neurons in the human brain.

MYTH NUMBER 14: IT'S ALL DOWNHILL ONCE YOU HIT YOUR '20S

Earlier, we talked about fluid intelligence that we associated with decline after peaking at the age of 18. We also mentioned that, apart from fluid intelligence, there is also mental intelligence which gets better as you age. Research suggests that to some extent, you actually become smarter, apart from becoming wiser with age (Brodwin, 2016). It is essential to note that your ability to use a more complex vocabulary and do basic math tends to continue improving until you reach 50 years of age. Of note is also the fact that your ability to recall recent events and reading the emotions of others do not begin to dwindle until after 30 years of age.

MYTH NUMBER 15: YOU'RE BORN WITH ALL THE BRAIN CELLS YOU'LL EVER HAVE

If you recall well, we talked about the hippocampus and neurogenesis earlier. Research has helped a lot in dismissing the myth that you are born with all the brain cells that you will ever have. According to a team of Swedish scientists in 1998, the hippocampus is able to continue creating new memories and to produce new neurons, even into old age (Brodwin, 2016). In 2014, another team of Swedish scientists revealed that new brain cells can also be formed in the striatum, which is responsible for motor control, decision-making, and motivation.

MYTH NUMBER 16: THE SO-CALLED *AHA!* MOMENTS ARE RARE AND RANDOM

The truth is that *Aha!* moments are not rare and random. According to a recent study, there is a location in the brain where these moments tend to take place. The neuroscientists that were carrying out the research studied creativity and insight for around 10 years and emphasized that the so-called *eureka* moments always happen. It has also been revealed that these

Aha! moments normally result from the same creative process that may eventually lead to a new concept or idea.

MYTH NUMBER 17: DRUGS CREATE HOLES IN YOUR BRAIN

It is true that drugs are capable of producing immediate remarkable effects when you take them. However, in the long term, taking drugs may cause you to develop unwanted side effects. Read on to find out if these side effects include the creation of holes in your brain.

It has been noted that drugs do not drill physical holes in the brain but they have a way of interfering with the brain chemistry. In fact, substances such as heroin cause alterations in the levels of neurotransmitters in the brain. In cases where someone abuses heroin, the drug is converted into morphine when it reaches the brain. The result is that an individual's motivational system gets hijacked by way of attachment to special receptors, thereby affecting one's perception of pain and rewards. With this information, it is now clear that the notion about drugs creating holes in your brain is merely a myth.

MYTH NUMBER 18: MALE BRAINS ARE MORE LOGICAL, FEMALE BRAINS ARE MORE EMPATHETIC

Owing to the fact that there are minor anatomical variations between the brains of males and females, one may subsequently think that there are also some slight variations in the way they think. However, no particular differences in ability have been linked to the anatomical variations. Cultural expectations have been pinpointed as a result of the inherent gender-related differences. For instance, women are more likely to do better in comparison to men when it comes to empathy and emotional intelligence tests. In other instances, it has been noted that if test subjects are informed that men perform better, the men tend to actually exhibit improved performance or may perform as equally as women would do. Having said this, it is clear that saying that male brains are more logical, female brains are more empathetic is indeed a myth.

MYTH NUMBER 19: YOU ONLY HAVE FIVE SENSES

You may be extremely taken aback to hear that it is a myth that you only have five senses. This is because the five senses are the most talked about from childhood, growing up. It is interesting to note that there are other senses that we possess.

Did you know that you have a sense of balance that is in your inner ear? This sense is also referred to as your internal GPS or equilibrioception. It is responsible for telling you if you are lying down, sitting, or standing. You also have a sense of pain called nociception and a sense of where your body parts are located and what actions they are doing called proprioception. In addition to these senses, you also have thermoreception, which is a sense of temperature. There is also another sense called chronoception, which is involved in the passage of time. The other sense that humans have is interoception, which is mostly about internal needs such as needing to utilize the bathroom, thirst, or hunger. With all these senses, we can dismiss the myth that you only have five senses.

MYTH NUMBER 20: IF YOU LOSE A NEURAL PATHWAY, YOU NEVER GET IT BACK

It is possible to lose a neural pathway and get it back. Some people believe that once you lose a neural pathway, it is impossible for you to get it back. It is possible to restore and even further develop neural pathways that had been deactivated (Kulmo, 2019). There are only a few connections that cannot be re-established once they are lost. Simply put, it is correct to say that you have many opportunities to learn new things even as you age. On that note, it is incorrect to say that if you lose a neural pathway, you never get it back.

MYTH NUMBER 21: CHILDREN NEED ENRICHED LEARNING ENVIRONMENTS

It is a misconception to say that children need enriched learning environments. This misconception stems from a rat experiment that was carried out in a certain study. In the experiment, it was found that rats that were placed in empty cages had weaker cognitive development than those in big cages which had numerous stimuli like climbing poles and exercise wheels. The results from the rat experiment were incorrectly interpreted to have a meaning in relation to children.

Results obtained from the study exclusively showed the reaction of rats not that of human children. It has been noted that children are highly skillful and teachable. Therefore, there is no need for them to be exposed to "brain tools." However, this does not mean that parents should not provide their children with the appropriate toys if need be. The truth is that under normal growth conditions, children are able to encounter the necessary stimuli that they need for proper learning and development.

MYTH NUMBER 22: YOU CAN TRAIN YOUR BRAIN TO BE SMARTER

It is partially true to say that you can train your brain to be smarter. Please note that keeping your brain active is remarkable. However, it is possible that you may be good at using your brain to solve certain problems but you may also find that other tasks may be difficult for you to deal with. Learning to do something new and breaking your everyday routine are possible actions and actually good for the brain. Nevertheless, these actions may not be successful in training your brain to be smarter.

MYTH NUMBER 23: CORTISOL IS A STRESS HORMONE AND SEROTONIN IS A HAPPINESS HORMONE

The hormone cortisol is normally associated with stress whereas serotonin is linked to happiness. However, it should be understood that each and every hormone does not have a singular psychological purpose. All the chemicals that are involved in the creation of your mind work together. For instance, according to your brain's needs, cortisol is able to boost glucose levels in your bloodstream so that energy is provided to your cells whether or not you feel stressed. Prior to awakening in the morning or just before you engage in exercise, your brain is able to convey signals to your adrenal glands so that they can release cortisol. Clearly, cortisol can be released during stressful conditions, but it is not a "stress hormone."

In the same manner, you should note that serotonin is not a happiness hormone. It has numerous functions. For example, serotonin is responsible for keeping track of your energy gain and expenditure in your brain. Serotonin also functions to control the amount of fat that is made in your body. The other function of serotonin is to permit you to utilize energy even when an immediate reward is unavailable such as when you are curious or you want to explore. Serotonin is also involved in assisting other neurons to do a back-and-forth communication process when it comes to the creation of thoughts, actions, perceptions, and feelings. It is clear now that it is incorrect to say that cortisol is a stress hormone and serotonin is a happiness hormone.

MYTH NUMBER 24: YOUR BRAIN REACTS TO THE EVENTS IN THE WORLD

Your brain seems to be reacting to events that occur throughout the day. It is important to note that your brain is in a constant state of guessing what could possibly happen in the next moment. In addition to making these guesses, the brain compares them with the sense data that emanates from the external world as well as inside your body. These guesses act as the seeds that are responsible for producing your resultant actions and experiences.

By the time your brain receives sense data from your nose, eyes or other parts of your body, your brain will have already identified these actions. Just as if it is a fortune teller, your brain keeps on predicting, imagining, or in a sense, wondering what will happen to you. The interesting phenomena about these actions of the brain are very rapid and effortless such that you will feel as if you are reacting. Therefore, the myth that your brain reacts to events in the world can safely be dismissed.

MYTH NUMBER 25: MIRROR NEURONS ARE SPECIAL CELLS THAT CREATE EMPATHY

According to a study that was carried out a number of decades ago, some researchers observed neurons that seemed as if they possessed a specific type of symmetry. These neurons were believed to increase their activity when a particular action was taken. Such actions included waving your hand or in some instances, watching others carry out a similar action. Simply because of this unique behavior of theirs, these neurons were referred to as "mirror neurons." However, in truth, they are merely everyday neurons that are involved in normal, miraculous predictions.

Bear in mind that predictions start as silent commands to perform certain movements of your body parts. Following these predictions, copies of commands are then sent to your sensory systems so that actual actions are seen, heard, or felt if there is a movement. These commands may or may not be executed, but they are an important part of your capability to perceive anything, even other people's actions. Simply put, the same neurons may help you to carry out different forms of actions that fall into the same category. For example, waving or wiggling fingers as a way of greeting some-one. Clearly, it's not "mirroring" but a normal predic-tive process of your brain. Therefore, it is indeed a myth to say that mirror neurons are special cells that create empathy.

CONCLUSION

A happier life is highly linked to the health of your brain, even in the later years of your existence. It is possible to remain smart, with excellent information retaining and recalling acumen during your golden days. This book is an effective compilation of practical strategies for keeping your brain healthy and sound, regardless of the circumstances.

Your brain is one of the most complex organs, with various parts that are responsible for different functions. Some of the important components are the hippocampus, cerebral cortex, brain stem, cerebrum, and cerebellum. As you age, the brain naturally goes through structural, chemical, neuronal, and cognitive changes. While there are a few people who can escape these changes, there are options to slow the progression through healthy lifestyle choices. Eating healthy, exercising, and sleeping well, in addition to creating and sustaining meaningful relationships are some of the tips that were emphasized in this book.

Eating foods such as avocados, oranges, broccoli, and eggs will boost the health of your brain. Even the simplest exercise will see your brain developing more neural networks and becoming more effective in its functions. It is also recommended that when you sleep, you should get into a deep sleep for at least seven hours. Sleeping gives your busy brain some time to rest, thereby rejuvenating it. Create as many opportunities for interacting with others as much as possible. Attend meetings, join support groups, and call friends and relatives, just to mention a few. Finding a purpose in life is linked to neuroplasticity and better brain health. Interestingly, the things that can foster happiness in your life are very simple, yet they are easy to neglect. Identify what makes you happy and go for it.

This book ends by listing various myths that have become so grounded to the extent that many people think they are true. This helps to free you from being misled by such baseless statements. One of such myths is that you can never have more brain cells than the ones that you are born with. On the contrary, you can develop more brain cells and neural networks as time progresses. Most of us have always been told that once you reach your twenties, your brain begins to deteriorate, no matter what you do. This is another myth, considering that interventions such as working out can keep your brain active and effective.

I really hope that this book gives you insights that boost your confidence with regard to taking good care of your brain. You can be the next *super-ager* of your time if you put the recommendations that were mentioned in this book into practice. Happy super-aging!

AUTHOR BIOGRAPHY

Walter Bishop moved to Eritrea at the age of four, then to Sweden until the age of eight. He then grew up in New York where he has lived all his life. Bishop is the youngest child of six siblings and is now a father of two. He has always been curious about brain development and human behavior, starting from his teen years when his father developed dementia. The author saw how the whole family helped to take care of his father.

Considering that dementia can be inherited, Bishop actively sought knowledge on how he can counteract or delay the process and effects of the aging brain so that he would be independent for as long as possible and avoid burdening his family to the greatest extent. His knowledge and experience in the area make him an authority on the subject of maintaining an aging brain and he wants to share what he knows with others who can benefit from it. Bishop has a practical testimony that the nuggets that are given in this book do work because they have contributed to notable changes in his life. What he has discovered is that the preventive work done on the brain has a long-lasting effect later in life.

Bishop wants to share his knowledge on brain development and human behavior with readers who need the information. He hopes this book can help the readers have a healthier outlook on life.

REFERENCES

Ackerman, C. (2018, July 25). *What is neuroplasticity? A psychologist explains [+14 exercises].* Positive Psych https://positivepsychology.com/neuroplasticity/

Berkman, L. F., & Syme, S. L. (1979). Social networks, host resistance, and mortality: A nine-year follow-up study of Alameda County residents. *American Journal of Epidemiology, 109*(2), 186–204. https://doi.org/10.1093/oxfordjournals.aje.a112674

Bonakdarpour, B. (2022). *10 surprising facts about your brain.* Northwestern Medicine. https://www.nm.org/healthbeat/healthy-tips/ten-surprising-facts-about-your-brain

Brodwin, E. (2016, March 22). *11 common myths about the brain that need to be smashed.* Business Insider. https://www.businessinsider.com/myths-about-the-brain-2016-3

Centers for Disease Prevention and Control. (2019, March 25). *Subjective cognitive decline—A public health issue.* CDC. https://www.cdc.gov/aging/data/subjective-cognitive-decline-brief.html

Cherry, K. (2012, July 2). *Phineas Gage's brain injury.* Verywell well. https://www.verywellmind.com/phineas-gage-2795244

Cherry, K. (2020, May 15). *What is memory and how does it work?* Verywell well. https://www.verywellmind.com/what-is-memory-2795006

Cherry, K. (2021, September 9). *7 myths about the brain debunked.* Verywell Mind. https://www.verywellmind.com/myths-about-the-brain-2794884

Cherry, K. (2022, February 18). *How our brain neurons can change over time from life's experience.* Verywell Mind. https://www.verywellmind.com/what-is-brain-plasticity-2794886

Chui, H. (1996). Alzheimer Disease. *Alzheimer disease and associated disorders, 10*(1), 53. https://doi.org/10.1097/00002093-199603000-00009

Clearvue Health. (2019, June 27). *A Sense of Purpose Helps You Live Longer*. Clearvue Health. https://www.clearvuehealth.com/b/purpose-longevity-health/

Cleveland Clinic. (n.d.). *6 pillars of brain health: Social interaction*. Healthy Brains by Cleveland Clinic. https://healthybrains.org/pillar-social/

Damasio, A. (2014). *USC Dana and David Dornsife College of Letters, Arts and Sciences*. Usc.edu. https://dornsife.usc.edu/cf/faculty-and-staff/faculty.cfm?pid=1008328

Ebert, A. R., Kulibert, D., & McFadden, S. H. (2019). Effects of dementia knowledge and dementia fear on comfort with people having dementia: Implications for dementia-friendly communities. *Dementia*, 147130121982770. https://doi.org/10.1177/1471301219827708

Evans, K. (2018, September 17). *Why relationships are the key to longevity*. Mindful. https://www.mindful.org/why-relationships-are-the-key-to-longevity/

Feldman-Barrett, L. (2021, May 28). *7 (and a half) myths about your brain*. BBC Science Focus Magazine. https://www.sciencefocus.com/the-human-body/7-and-a-half-myths-about-your-brain/

Gunnars, K. (2021, October 25). *Mediterranean Diet 101: A meal plan and beginner's guide*. Healthline; Healthline Media. https://www.healthline.com/nutrition/mediterranean-diet-meal-plan

Healthwise Staff. (n.d.). *Social connections*. Myhealth.alberta.ca. https://myhealth.alberta.ca/health/Pages/conditions.aspx?hwid=abl0295&

Hopper, E. (2020, July 28). *How your social life might help you live longer*. Greater Good. https://greatergood.berkeley.edu/article/item/how_your_social_life_might_help_you_life_longer

Huberman Lab. (2021, December 22). *5 steps to enhance quality of connection with yourself and others during the holidays and new year*. Huberman Lab. https://hubermanlab.com/5-steps-to-enhance-quality-of-connection-with-yourself-and-others-during-the-holidays-and-new-year/

Huberman, A. (2021, October 29). *Teach and learn better with a "neuroplasticity super protocol."* Huberman Lab. https://hubermanlab.com/teach-and-learn-better-with-a-neuroplasticity-super-protocol/

Jennings, K.-A. (2021, June 4). *11 best foods to boost your brain and memory*. Healthline. https://www.healthline.com/nutrition/11-brain-foods

John Hopkins Medicine. (2019). *Anatomy of the brain*. Johns Hopkins Medicine. https://www.hopkinsmedicine.org/health/conditions-and-diseases/anatomy-of-the-brain

John Hopkins Medicine. (2022). *Keep your brain young with music*. Hopkins Medicine. https://www.hopkinsmedicine.org/health/wellness-and-prevention/keep-your-brain-young-with-music

Kulmo, W. M. (2019, February 12). *Eight myths about your brain*. Norwegian SciTech News. https://norwegianscitechnews.com/2019/02/eight-myths-about-your-brain/

Mayo Clinic Staff. (2021, July 23). *Mediterranean diet: A heart-healthy eating plan*. Mayo Clinic. https://www.mayoclinic.org/healthy-lifestyle/nutrition-and-healthy-eating/in-depth/mediterranean-diet/art-20047801

Mayo Clinic Staff. (2022). *How to make the DASH diet work for you*. Mayo Clinic. https://www.mayoclinic.org/healthy-lifestyle/nutrition-and-healthy-eating/in-depth/dash-diet/art-20048456

McDermott, K. B. (2013). *Memory (encoding, storage, retrieval)*. Noba. https://nobaproject.com/modules/memory-encoding-storage-retrieval

Medicine, N. (2019, October). *11 Fun facts about your brain*. Northwestern Medicine. https://www.nm.org/healthbeat/healthy-tips/11-fun-facts-about-your-brain

Migala, J. (2020, November 2). *What is the Mediterranean diet? Food list, meal plan, benefits*. Everyday Health. https://www.everydayhealth.com/mediterranean-diet/guide/

Nagasawa, M., Mitsui, S., En, S., Ohtani, N., Ohta, M., Sakuma, Y., Onaka, T., Mogi, K., & Kikusui, T. (2015). Oxytocin-gaze positive loop and the coevolution of human-dog bonds. *Science, 348*(6232), 333–336. https://doi.org/10.1126/science.1261022

Nichols, H. (2020, September 9). *What happens to the brain as we age?* Medical News Today. https://www.medicalnewstoday.com/articles/319185

NIH. (n.d.). *Brain Basics: The life and death of a neuron.* National Institute of Neurological Disorders and Stroke. https://www.ninds.nih.gov/health-information/patient-caregiver-education/brain-basics-life-and-death-neuron

Northwestern Medicine. (2022). *10 surprising facts about your brain.* Northwestern Medicine. https://www.nm.org/healthbeat/healthy-tips/ten-surprising-facts-about-your-brain

Novotney, A. (2022). *The real secrets to a longer life.* Apa.org. https://www.apa.org/monitor/2011/12/longer-life

Palmer, K., Fratiglioni, L., & Winblad, B. (2003). What is mild cognitive impairment? Variations in definitions and evolution of nondemented persons with cognitive impairment. *Acta Neurologica Scandinavica,* *107,* 14–20. https://doi.org/10.1034/j.1600-0404.107.s179.2.x

Parker-Pope, T. (2022, January 24). The best brain foods you're not eating. *The New York Times.* https://www.nytimes.com/2022/01/24/well/eat/brain-food.html

Paul, M. (2008, November 18). *"Super" ager brains reveal first secrets of sharp memory in old age.* Northwestern University News. https://www.northwestern.edu/newscenter/stories/2008/11/superaged.html

Rettner, R. (2013, September 25). *Busted! Most in US believe brain disease myths.* Live Science. https://www.livescience.com/39923-americans-believe-brain-myths.html

Rice, A. (2022, April 22). *Can a purpose-driven life improve brain health? New research says yes.* Psych Central. https://psychcentral.com/news/life-purpose-linked-to-better-brain-health

Saints, E. (n.d.). *J.Lo Proved On SNL (Again) That she's aging backwards - Here are some of her beauty secrets.* Eight Saints. https://eightsaintsskincare.com/blogs/page-eight/j-lo-proved-on-snl-again-that-she-s-aging-backwards-here-are-some-of-her-beauty-secrets

Sandoiu, A. (2018, August 1). *Do brain-training games really work?* Medical News Today.com. https://www.medicalnewstoday.com/articles/322648

Seppala, E. (2014, May 9). *Connectedness and health: The science of social connection*. The Center for Compassion and Altruism Research and Education. http://ccare.stanford.edu/uncategorized/connected ness-health-the-science-of-social-connection-infographic/

Singer, E. (2021, September 14). *Super agers and centenarians: The search for protective factors*. Simons Foundation. https://www.simonsfoun dation.org/2021/09/14/super-agers-and-centenarians-the-search-for-protective-factors/

Spielman, R. M., Dumper, K., Jenkins, W., Lacombe, A., Lovett, M., & Perlmutter, M. (2014, December 8). *Parts of the brain involved with memory*. OpenStax. https://opentextbc.ca/psychologyopenstax/chapter/parts-of-the-brain-involved-with-memory/

Sreenivas, S. (2021, September 27). *What to know about the MIND Diet*. WebMD. https://www.webmd.com/alzheimers/what-to-know-about-mind-diet

GCBH recommendations on social engagement and brain health. (n.d.). https://www.aarp.org/content/dam/aarp/health/brain_health/2017/02/gcbh-social-engagement-report-english-aarp.doi.10.26419%252Fpia.00015.001.pdf

UCSF Magazine. (n.d.). *Decoding the mystery of the super-ager. UCSF Magazine*. https://magazine.ucsf.edu/decoding-mystery-super-ager

Villines, Z. (2021, August 11). *The serious effects of alcohol on the brain*. WebMD. https://www.webmd.com/connect-to-care/addiction-treatment-recovery/alcohol/serious-effects-alcohol-on-brain

Virtues for life.com. (2022, April 29). *6 benefits of having a sense of purpose*. https://www.virtuesforlife.com/6-benefits-of-having-a-sense-of-purpose-infographic/

WebMD Editorial Contributors. (2021, March 29). *What to know about foods for brain health*. WebMD. https://www.webmd.com/brain/what-to-know-about-foods-for-brain-health

Wikipedia Contributors. (2019a, February 21). *Decay theory*. Wikipedia; Wikimedia Foundation. https://en.wikipedia.org/wiki/Decay_theory

Wikipedia Contributors. (2019b, December 17). *Interference theory*. Wikipedia; Wikimedia Foundation. https://en.wikipedia.org/wiki/Interference_theory

Wnuk, A. (2019). *How the brain changes with age.* Brainfacts.org. https://www.brainfacts.org/thinking-sensing-and-behaving/aging/2019/how-the-brain-changes-with-age-083019

Woodruff, A. (2016, November 22). *What is a neuron?* Qbi.uq.edu.au. https://qbi.uq.edu.au/brain/brain-anatomy/what-neuron

Wright, K. C. (2018, June). *Mediterranean diet improves cognition, memory, and brain volume.* Today's Dietitian Magazine.. https://www.todays dietitian.com/newarchives/0618p40.shtml

IMAGE REFERENCES

Anatomy of a typical human neuron. Structure neuron. (n.d.). IStock. Retrieved July 13, 2022, from https://www.istockphoto.com/se/vektor/structure-of-a-motor-neuron-gm534025955-56400452?clarity=false

Profile view of a human brain. Cartoon vector illustration for... (n.d.). IStock. Retrieved July 13, 2022, from https://www.istockphoto.com/se/vektor/human-brain-illustration-gm494790922-77653189?clarity=false

9 789198 840605